CW00543417

Cover design by Eleanor Perkins
Cover images by Pexels, Canva.com

Sketches – Copyright © 2021 Laura Perkins

Printed by Book Printing UK

Written and printed during the COVID-19 pandemic

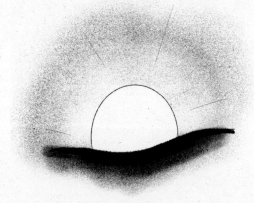

LETTERS TO
OTHER WOMEN

Let's Talk About It

For Ruth and Dee,
my 'Yardley Girls'

And for my mother, Maggie,
to whom I am extremely grateful.
You are a wonderful woman.

"*Anything that's human is mentionable, and anything that is mentionable can be more manageable. When we talk about our feelings, they become less overwhelming, less upsetting, and less scary. The people we trust with that important talk can help us know that we are not alone*"

Words from Fred Rogers,
American TV Presenter and Writer

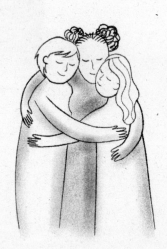

Let's Talk About It

I'd like to thank you for picking up this book. Whether you've grabbed it quickly because it mentions miscarriage and you desperately don't want to feel alone; whether you've yet to embark on your journey and want to flick through the pages to be better informed; or whether indeed you are one of the marvellous and brave women who have contributed to its pages and want to caress your own words on the page. Thank you.

The idea for the book has been floating around in my mind for some time. On a personal level, I have struggled with fertility; 2 years 3 months of trying and peeing on sticks to finally create my son and another 3 years of trying for his sibling.

As naive youngsters, we're prepared so much for contraception and the biology of periods, conception and birth, but we don't talk enough about the struggles of trying to get pregnant, the heartache of losing a baby during pregnancy or if a baby is born sleeping. I am a teacher and often have the opportunity to sit in on PSHE lessons, listening to the nurses discuss pregnancy and conception. In a recent lesson, our nurse explained how easy it was to get pregnant. "No it's bloody not!" I shouted, brandishing my ovulation app. Twenty teen heads turn around to stare as I continue my rant, "I ovulated on Saturday, had sex 3 times that day alone, necked the bottle of folic acid and I'm still as barren as the desert!" I started to weep.

I of course then snapped out of my daydream as one of the kids started blowing up a condom. Instead, I sat there silently seething, knowing that one of them was bound to get up the duff before I did.

It's difficult to discuss personal problems and all things Woman in the workplace. I have only started to pluck up the courage to talk to my close colleagues about my fertility issues, and in fact any 'woman' issues. Shame and Guilt have pinned me to my desk and taped my mouth shut in the past. I recently read 'It's About Bloody Time' by Emma Barnett and it got me thinking of all the women who are shuffling around their offices, power-walking along corridors stuffing tampons in pockets and sanitary pads in bras. Listen up, people: Women have periods. And women miscarry. They give birth to children who have already died. They struggle to get pregnant. They suffer from unbelievably awful periods. They take multiple drugs to help IVF treatment. Why on Earth are we not talking about this more? I'm not saying that the AOB on the weekly agenda should be menstruation and miscarriage, or that we should wave around ovulation sticks in those lucky 24-hour windows, but should we not normalise these conversations?

This stuff can be earth-shattering, soul-destroying, and all-consuming. It affects mental health, relationships, work and family. We shouldn't be talking in hushed tones in a corner, hoping no-one checking the CCTV can lip read.

So, during the pandemic, and after starting to come to terms with my 'dream' not becoming a reality, (incidentally the book The Next Happy by Tracey Cleantis will help anyone whose Dream is essentially over) I decided to collect a whole range of stories, or 'letters', from real women about their periods, fertility, pregnancies, loss, and successes and for others to see that no-one is alone in fighting a battle that - for many - is a silent one, but that so many of us share.

These letters aren't 'to women' because we're making a feminist or sexist statement. Men were welcomed to contribute to this project but none came forward. This time. Before women open up to wider circles, line managers and employers, they should feel confident in discussing details of their lives with peers, friends and like-minded women. This project hopefully provides the opportunity to begin this process. The men mentioned in this book are celebrated and I hope that you are able to invite the men in your own lives to share these stories with you.

I wanted each contribution to be real, honest, but ideally hopeful; what has been learnt along the way, what has changed, what help has been given/taken? I hope you take comfort in the suggestions and ideas in these sections. Get out your best highlighters and favourite notebook to scribble down some inspiration.

I have learnt so much about these women: (I consider some of them my closest friends, others I've only met through this project) the pain they have carried; the anxieties they experience daily; the brutal brushes with professionals they've had to endure; the medical procedures they have had. I've learnt from them that I'm not alone in my fear of 'the white coat'; I have realised that 1 in 4 pregnancies end in miscarriage (stat confirmed by Tommy's); I know what signs to look out for during miscarriage and what I will have to consider afterwards; I have learnt that there is hope, and success; I've learnt that sometimes there isn't and that is manageable too.

This book won't shy away from detail, it won't skip the bits with blood in or pretend that life carried on a few days later. But that's what I'm looking for. Raw, open, honest. Real women's voices sharing a sense of fact, detail, humour, solemnity...whatever has worked best for them to get their letter on the page. These were collected at various stages during the COVID pandemic of 2020 and by the time this comes to print, I know that circumstances will have changed for several women.

I've added a little introduction to each woman (who appear in alphabetical order) which sums up their experience, just in case you are not quite ready to delve into their experience yet, or of course if there are certain ones that you yearn to read first.

I know many of these wonderful women found the process cathartic as they wrote their words. I hope you find support, reassurance and guidance in this book. It's definitely time to Talk About It.

Periods
Lottie
Emily

Polycystic Ovary Syndrome
Chrissy
Nicole
Rebekah
Shareena

Endometriosis
Anais
Emily (undiagnosed)
Naomi
Tamara

Ovarian Torsion
Becky

Single Ovary
Marlene

Low Egg Count
Ellie

Infertility
Beki
Ellie

Secondary Infertility
Lell
Leonie

Intrauterine insemination
Ellie
Lil

Intracytoplasmic sperm injection
Shareena

Donor Sperm
Helen

In Vitro Fertilisation
Ellie
Helen
Leonie
Lil
Lucy

Miscarriage
Amy
Cate
Chrissy
Dee
Jane
Lorna
Nicole

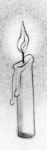

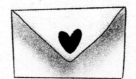

Amy

Amy was told she was 'silly' after her first miscarriage but was treated much better after her second. Here she explains that it's best to be open and honest.

My name is Amy and I am 31. I live in mid-Wales and am a part-time special needs teacher. The rest of the week I am at home with my 2 sons – Rowan who is 5 and Lewi who has just turned 3. I have had 2 miscarriages and had a very different experience each time.

The first time I was 22 and the pregnancy was very much unplanned. I had a copper coil fitted and my periods whilst using it were erratic and/ or absent. It never even crossed my mind that I could be pregnant. I was at home one evening when I suddenly had pain in my lower abdomen, just on the one side. It felt like someone had run me through with a hot poker and the pain took my breath away. I was also bleeding heavily so I rang ShropDoc who suspected an ectopic pregnancy. I was in total shock. As far as I was concerned I had had a (very light) period a few weeks ago. We're talking a couple of days of light spotting – I had just counted myself lucky and thought no more of it. I later learned (from Dr Google) that this was more than likely implantation bleeding which I had never even heard of at that point. I did a pregnancy test which showed as positive and went to the GP the following morning. They sent me to the hospital for a scan later the same day.

I had scans to determine the location of the foetus (not ectopic) and then blood tests every other day for 14 days to track the hormone levels. They were meant to be going down but they plateau-ed and then rose slightly in the middle of that time. They were unsure what was going on so I was in a sort of limbo or a while - feeling shocked and terrified of either possible outcome: a miscarriage or a viable pregnancy.

The actual medical processes were fine and quite efficient but the attitudes towards me from doctors and midwives were... indifferent at best, unkind at worst. There was a definite implication from the way I was spoken to that what I was going through mattered less than those women who were older/had planned to be pregnant. When they finally came to the conclusion that I had miscarried I wasn't taken to a private area and spoken to kindly. A very brusque doctor came to me in a waiting area in a corridor and literally said "There is no baby. Go home." She then turned to walk away without offering any opportunity to ask any questions. Luckily my mother had come to the hospital with me that day. If I had been on my own/just with my partner I probably would have just done as I was told. She demanded to speak to someone properly. The doctor rolled her eyes at us and said we could wait and she would talk to us "if she had time". We waited nearly 3 hours to speak to her again and she was so cold and uncaring. She even called me "silly" when I became upset. I totally appreciate that many people have miscarriages and they don't always have the answers but to totally shut down the opportunity to ask made me feel awful.

Whatever she said, I can say for absolute certainty that there was a baby of some level of development (whether it was technically classed as an embryo or a foetus, I don't know). I know because I passed pieces of it at home later on, including a tiny hand with partially formed fingers. This was obviously quite traumatic and has always made me wonder whether I was further along than I thought at the time, as I have read more about foetal development since.

I'm quite a pragmatic person so for a long time afterwards I just got on with life. I moved to Bristol and started a totally new job a few months, which when I look back I can see was probably catalysed by the miscarriage. A while later I read some research that detailed how taking ibuprofen in early pregnancy significantly increases the risk of miscarriage. At the time of my first miscarriage, I had been taking the maximum dose of it for at least a fortnight after an injury at work. I would never have taken a single tablet had I had any inkling that I might be pregnant. That information hit me really hard and I felt quite down and guilty for a while. Although it hadn't been part of my plan at that time, had it been a viable pregnancy I would have made it work. I was in a stable relationship and job so I would have had no reason not to, in my view.

My support at this time was mostly ranting to my partner or my mum when I became overwhelmed (or had too much to drink). There was absolutely no support offered by the doctor/midwives. Not even a pamphlet. In time, I came to see that it wasn't my fault and I didn't knowingly harm the baby. I do still feel guilty about it now when I think about it too much though.

Five years later, I had another miscarriage. This one was between two successful pregnancies with my 2 sons. This time I was 27, married and the baby was very much planned. My physical symptoms were much more subtle this time (backache and light spotting to begin with) and I already knew I was pregnant. I knew it was happening as soon as I saw the first spot of blood. I remember going to Morrison's and buying a digital test in their toilets (I couldn't wait until I drove the half-hour home) which showed up as "pregnant – 2 weeks". The previous week another test had said "pregnant – 3+ weeks" so I knew the hormone levels were already dropping. When I went to the hospital for a scan and was told there was no heartbeat the attitudes from staff were completely different from the first time around. There was a lot of compassion, care and reassurance. Whether that was because I was in a different stage and situation in life or just due to encountering different staff, I can't say for sure. All I know is that I was treated very, very differently.

When I had the second miscarriage I was far more open with friends and colleagues which I guess comes with age and life experience. Also, I was already a part of a Facebook group made up of women who all got married around the same time as me. It started as a wedding planning group then evolved into something else. Some of the women have gone on to have babies, some haven't. Some have struggled with infertility and loss, some haven't.

I have learned a lot about the struggles many people go through concerning pregnancy and parenthood. The main thing they have in common is that they are all incredibly supportive of one another. I have come to regard them as friends, despite never having met any of them in real life. I would definitely recommend finding a similar group to anyone.

www.facebook.com/amyltraylor

Anais

Anais has yet to begin her path to pregnancy, but is already facing the problems she may encounter. Endometriosis has taken Anais to a dark place but as you'll see from her story, she has emerged happy and hopeful.

I'm 22 years old, and just about to start my Masters in Translation Studies after a 4-year degree in French and Translation. I absolutely love my course, and I'm working hard to become a medical translator. I have lovely friends and a fantastic university, but I struggled in silence for years with something I did not even tell my best friends about until things got out of hand.

At college, I was put on hormones to control my irregular periods, and for a couple of years, I was constantly swapping pills. One gave me severe migraines, the other gave me acne, the other made my periods worse, etc. etc. The usual problems women and girls have on the pill. During my first year of uni, I decided that enough was enough, and I came off birth control altogether. I knew there was no risk of me getting pregnant (I'm a lesbian) and I'd convinced myself by that point that things couldn't possibly be worse if I came off them (ohhhh was I wrong!). Suffering from depression that I thought could be related to the pill, I stopped taking it, and one month later is when all my lovely problems started.

A few days after moving back home for the summer, I had excruciating pain in my stomach. I was in so much pain that paracetamol and ibuprofen did nothing at all. I was sat on the kitchen floor with a bucket thinking I'd eaten a dodgy piece of chicken, hoping it would pass. Three days later and still in agony, I dragged myself to the doctors.

'Are you currently on your period?'

'Yes', I said.

'It's probably just period pain. Take some paracetamol and do some gentle exercise.' Had I really just gone to the doctors to be told a couple of sit-ups was going to solve my problems?

My entire summer holidays were spent lying on the sofa with a hot water bottle and a constant supply of paracetamol. Nothing helped. Whenever I ate food, my stomach would hurt so much that I would sit and cry at the table. My parents were worried and didn't know what to suggest. My appetite disappeared, I hardly ate, and I became even more unhappy. I saw the doctor a few more times, and I was given peppermint capsules to aid digestion and told it was probably IBS. They said there was nothing to do but take paracetamol whenever I had pain, and to watch out for certain trigger foods.

Going back to uni in the second year was difficult. I was severely unhappy, and my pain was stopping me from going out and enjoying myself. Throughout the second year, I was put on many different birth control pills again for my irregular periods which, surprise surprise, had come back again – I would have no period for two months, then a period that lasted three weeks. With every period the pain in my abdomen returned, and no doctor seemed to think my pain was abnormal.

'Have you tried the low FODMAP diet?' They suggested, after I had been on a strict low FODMAP diet for a year by then.

'Have you tried exercising?' He asks me after I had been doing Taekwon-Do three times a week.

Then came my year abroad. By this time I'd accepted this constant pain was my new norm, and that I'd be like this for the rest of my life. The first few months of my year abroad living with my grandparents started off relatively well, that is, until I came off my birth control again.

The winter of 2018/2019 was one of the worst times of my life. My pain increased tenfold and there were days where I was passing out on the floor of my en-suite bathroom because the pain was so bad. There were days where I bled so heavily for weeks that I wondered where it was even coming from. To quote Lee Evans, 'this is somebody else's, this!'

I was rushed to A&E after one doctor prodded my stomach and decided I had a ruptured appendix. Six hours and two scans later, the theory was debunked. I was sat hooked up to morphine while doctors scratched their heads. Those few hours hooked up to strong painkillers was the first time in months that I was completely pain-free. It was glorious, and I felt dangerously free. A day later, my pain had returned and I was back to lying on my bed wondering how I was going to get through my exams. I was constantly exhausted, I couldn't eat any food, I felt sick and waves of pain would come back every time I tried to eat. The pain was so excruciating and so constant most days of the week that my depression came back stronger than ever. I started to feel suicidal after years of constant, unbearable pain, and the hopelessness and desperation that I felt knowing that nobody could help me.

On several occasions, I would be sat in front of a doctor crying my eyes out, literally begging them to stop the pain. Yet, I was still brushed away. One night, I sat by the fire and googled painless ways to end my life. A couple of searches later, the shock of what I was doing hit me and I felt horrified. I called my amazing counsellor and he helped calm me down and told me they would eventually find the cause of my pain.

On the 17th of February 2020, my 22nd birthday, I had a gynaecology appointment at Hereford Hospital. The doctor and nurses kindly listened to what I had to say and, after more scans and tests, diagnosed me with endometriosis. Endometriosis is when endometrial tissue in the uterus grows elsewhere, and blood pools into the wrong areas of your abdomen, causing extreme pain and nausea that gets worse on your period. When I was diagnosed, I cried and cried and cried. I thanked them over and over again and a nurse hugged me as I sobbed into her shoulder, the relief of finally being listened to and having an explanation for my pain after years of being ignored overwhelming me. It turns out, the first few pills I'd been on at college and the first year of uni had been managing my endometriosis symptoms, so I didn't even realise I'd developed it until I came off them.

My mum, who was waiting for me outside, cried with me when I told her. We celebrated with drinks and, strangely, I was happy. You might think it weird to feel so elevated after a diagnosis, but for me, it saved my life. I was given the hormonal implant and since then I have had manageable levels of pain, and the dark place I was in has gone. I have regular flare-ups that can last several weeks, but knowing I will not have to live the rest of my life in that agonising pain is what gets me through them. I would like to have a child biologically one day; however, depending on how badly scarred my reproductive organs are, this may not be easy. Endometriosis causes fertility problems for a lot of women. It's not perfect; there is no cure and I will have pain for the rest of my life, but now it is manageable, and there is HOPE, SUPPORT and INFORMATION.

My message to anyone else who is having unexplained chronic pain is never to give up. I was going to the doctors weekly at one point, desperate to get referred to a specialist. Four arduous years later, it happened. I was finally understood and supported, and it changed my life. It takes on average ten years for a woman to be diagnosed with endometriosis, which is abhorrent. That is why we have to listen to women; they know their own body and they know when something isn't right. Keep fighting and never let someone tell you what you're experiencing isn't valid. I'm now about to graduate (well, what with the current COVID-19 situation it will probably be on a Zoom meeting or something) and I'm looking forward to enjoying my master's degree with support from my university on how to manage my chronic condition. I know that my family and friends will be there for me every step of the way, and I am so thankful.

Instagram @anais_banneville

Becky

Becky had an unexpected operation when she was travelling due to a cyst in her fallopian tube. The quick turn of events meant her plans for the future were changed overnight.

My name is Becky and I am 36 years old. I always saw myself in later life, married with 2 or 3 children. I have always been passionate about working with children so I completed a diploma in childcare and education straight from leaving school. I then took up roles within a nursery setting working my way up to become a room leader. When I was 22 years old, I felt it was time for me to take some well deserved time out and go travelling. I had planned to be gone for 1 year but after being gone for the majority of that time and falling in love with Australia, my partner, at the time, and I decided to apply for residency there. We carried on with the rest of our world travelling whilst the visas were being processed and then returned to Australia to live.

2 months into starting our new adventure everything changed. I started experiencing excruciating lower abdominal pain. I went to the hospital and not long after they sent me home as my pain subsided and then totally went.

A couple of days later, the pain was back and worse. I went back to the hospital and they scanned me and found I had a cyst on my fallopian tube. I was given medication for the pain and was told not to worry and to expect the cyst to either shrink by itself or pop, and that will be that.

Another couple of days passed and the pain just got worse. It was so painful that I couldn't walk, I had cold sweats, was vomiting and screaming in pain. My partner had to carry me to the car and took me back to the hospital. They wheeled me in and scanned me again, then decided to operate. I remember them saying not to worry but the cyst had since grown and they needed to remove it via keyhole surgery.

Unfortunately not long after getting set up in Australia, my partner and I started to drift apart so at this point I felt all alone in a hospital I didn't know and in a country where none of my family or friends could be there to support me.

They operated on me and I came around in the recovery room but not enough for the staff to first realise. I could hear them talking, mentioning something about an ovary. I was so sore, disoriented, alone and when I properly came around the first thing I asked was, What's happened? Am I OK? What's wrong?

I was told it's all ok, I'm ok, but once they started to operate, they realised I had what was called an Ovarian Torsion and needed an operation called Unilateral Salpingo-Oophorectomy. I didn't have a clue what they were talking about! They explained an Ovarian Torsion is when an ovary twists around the ligaments that hold it in place. This twisting can cut off blood flow to the ovary and fallopian tube and in my case, the cyst had caused this and they had to remove one of my ovaries and Fallopian tube as they were dead. Also not via keyhole but by cutting right across just above my pubic bone.

I cried. I cried and cried and cried. I just wanted my mum! I felt completely lost and I just wanted to be back home in Guernsey. I was on so many drugs that, to be honest, I was all over the place. Between my family, they got flights sorted for me the minute I was safe and able to fly home. My partner wasn't able to get his own visa so he had to be on mine. Because I was leaving, he then had to too. We broke up after that.

I had never known or heard of anyone going through what I had experienced. I felt ugly with having this large horrible scar. I was heartbroken at the thought of not being able to have my own children yet caring for others that do. I had 3 siblings and started resenting them all as they each had 2 children. I had friends that were sleeping around without the use of protection and remember feeling so angry that they all had healthy female organs, yet didn't appreciate what they had and that they could potentially cause harm at any time, even after what I had been through. I felt like part of me was taken away and I was stripped of being fully female and was left with a long ugly scar. I turned quite angry with myself and shut myself away from many people.

Back during the part where I was still in Australia and knew I was coming home but had to wait to be well enough, a mum from the nursery where I used to work, heard I was returning and contacted me asking if I would consider being their family nanny.

I knew this was a step I'd have to make and the sooner the better, as hard as it was. I started work as soon as the doctor gave me the all-clear and being welcomed into the family and giving them all I could was the beginning of moving forward. It took a little time but knowing I was enjoying the company of children again without resentment was comforting and heartwarming.

When my next period came, it was normal and I was pleased. I then thought I would have 1 every other month but that wasn't the case. My one ovary now compensates for the one no longer there. VERY ANNOYING!! My body now also produces lower estrogen levels which affect my skin on a monthly basis. ALSO VERY ANNOYING.

When it came to relationships, I was very wary. I wouldn't have sex with just anyone and refused sex until that person got tested for sexually transmitted diseases. I knew this isn't what I had previously ever had but with only having 1 ovary and 1 Fallopian tube, I was determined to do what I could to keep them safe.

After the operation, I was in denial to anyone who asked me if I wanted children of my own. This question always cut deep and hurt! By saying I didn't want one, it was easier for me to cope with rather than knowing the truth to whether I could or not.

I then met Jon, who is now my husband (nearly 11 yrs ago now!) I told him I didn't want children and knowing that he already had a son, I knew that this news would be fine. Our relationship grew and I felt loved, content, constantly happy, like this was the one. I felt I could fully trust in him. 3 years into our relationship, my view on having my own child started to change. I wanted to be a mum. I wanted a child with Jon. I wanted to see if this was something I/we could have together. This came as a bit of a shock to him. We discussed having a child and took a few months to decide if we were going to go down this route of trying. The answer was yes and straight away I started prepping my body with the necessary vitamins and minerals to help. I changed my diet, gave up all drinking, and focused on generally being as healthy as I could (not that I wasn't already healthy). I was so scared with what we could potentially be faced with. Any underlying issues or complications. All the heartache I have spent years trying to push down and hide away from. At the same time, I was so excited that I was in a position where I could finally have a family of my very own.

6 weeks later, I tested positive! I couldn't believe it! I was shaking and overwhelmed with this feeling I've never experienced before and the rest is history. I now have a beautiful healthy daughter, Olivia, who was born the day before her due date and weighed 6.5lbs. My life was complete and I am grateful every day for my happy ending.

I continued to nanny for the same family, being able to take Olivia to work with me until the boys grew old enough to start secondary school. I then changed to childminding where I could work from home, being able to care for Olivia along with other children and I haven't looked back. I love my life and all the children I get to spend time with.

It still hurts to take myself back to the problems and upset I was faced with for so many years. Unfortunately, I am unable to offer any help in where to go to seek advice to those who may need it and I still have never met anyone else who has had an ovarian torsion or a Unilateral Salpingo-Oophorectomy. But what I would like to share, is that my door is always open for anyone who may need help in this area and please know that you are still able to conceive, carry and give birth with no problems even if you only have 1 ovary and 1 fallopian tube and that for me, getting back into childcare and being around little ones that I love unconditionally, helped me 100% to move on in life.

Beki

Meet Beki, who thought she was 'broken' and almost ended her relationship because she and her husband couldn't conceive. A change in lifestyle helped her successfully get pregnant.

Hi I'm Beki, I'm 33 years old and currently living in Rutland. I have been with my husband for 11 years and married for 6 years, we Have a son Damien Whos 2.5 years old.

I started dating my husband in October 2009 and things went very fast. By new years day 2010 we were engaged and living together. After being together for 2 years we decided that we wanted to start trying for a family, I was 24 years old and my husband was 29. In 2011 I went to the doctors and planned our pregnancy journey, I had the implant removed and was told that it could take up to a year to conceive as my body needed to get back to normal after the implant.

I was really naive about getting pregnant and thought it would literally happen the next month, I was so sure it was going to happen that I went out and brought a nursery set and baby clothes.

Me and my husband decided we needed a fresh start so we moved away to the seaside, away from family, and got ourselves new jobs, this was a fresh start for us both and we finally wanted some answers as to why we weren't getting pregnant.

My periods had always been bad ever since I was 13, I would be in that much pain that I would hide away in bed for the first 3 days of my period, I couldn't move. This just became the norm for me and I didn't think anything of it. My life had become Ovulation sticks and negative tests, every month the same. We went to see a fertility specialist in a hospital who wanted to start with me and if I was 'normal' then my husband would go in for tests. It came back that I had possible Endometriosis, they gave me an internal scan which they could only find one ovary at that time. I was told to carry on trying and that it would happen naturally and if it didn't, to go back 2 years later to look into IVF. My heart was broken, I knew it wasn't going to be easy for us anymore. I tried silly products online to try and help us, I used ovulation sticks daily and started taking folic acid. In the summer of 2014 just 4 months before our wedding I had the faintest line on a pregnancy test, it was hardly there but I could see it. I didn't get excited because I wanted to see those big red lines to make sure it was real. I was sat in the garden reading a book when I had this massive shooting pain in my stomach area, I thought I was coming on my period as I was a few days late. This pain was different, it was more intense and painful. I just had this urge to push, push whatever was inside me out. I won't go into detail but I'm pretty sure I had a miscarriage although I never sought help or went to doctors after, I didn't realise it at the time but now I can see it was.

In 2016 things were becoming more serious about trying for a baby, we had been trying for 5 years now and were yet to ask for IVF. In 2017 I would be turning 30 and my husband would be 36. I could see my younger friends getting pregnant and my friends my age were on their 2nd and 3rd babies. people would ask me all the time when I was planning on having children and I would tell them "I hate children" just so they wouldn't talk to me about it. Not many people know about the struggles me and my husband went through.

Every month I would get excited about doing a test then cry when it came back negative. I used to stare at my pregnant friends, hating them for having something I couldn't have, something my body was designed to do but couldn't.

I decided to focus on me, I lost 3 stone of weight, I quit smoking, quit drinking and I felt amazing and so healthy. I had gone from slob to fitness freak. I had also had my tonsils removed at the age of 29 which made me feel amazing and healthy. I was on top of the world and was looking forward to my fitness adventures. Christmas came and me and hubby had the best Christmas just messing about, enjoying each other's company and we put baby-making to the back of our minds just for a few weeks though.

In January 2017 I was working away from my husband and I had one of the worst phone calls we had ever had. I knew how much he wanted a family and my body wasn't giving him that so I rang him and told him if he wanted to leave me and start a family with someone else then this was his chance. I told him it wasn't working with us and made it sound like I was so unhappy when really I just wanted him to be happy. He told me he would rather have me and just me than a family with someone else.

When I got home I realised I was 3 days late for my period, I knew the only way to start my period was to take a test so it could be negative then I could stop stressing.

It was the first time I had ever brought my own pregnancy test. (normally my husband gets them for me) I went home and did the test and within seconds these perfect bright red lines popped up. I thought I was dreaming, I kept saying to myself "I'm pregnant I'M PREGNANT" I fell to the floor crying my eyes out, and when I told my husband he went outside and cried and said, "Thank god because I thought I was broken".

The things that got me through the whole journey were my husband, my family, and a Facebook group I've been in for 6 years now. I'm not sure what helped me get pregnant if it was the weight loss, the no-smoking or just having fun and not thinking about making a baby. But it did happen. It just took a long time but he is so worth every year I waited. I'm hoping to start trying for another baby soon and I'm really anxious it will take me another 5 years. I know next time though I won't be as stressed and I won't put so much pressure on myself as I did with Damien.

Cate

Here Cate tells us the brutal truth of suddenly not being pregnant and everything being over very quickly. Having a medical background helped her accept what happened.

Hi, I'm Cate. I'm 39 (almost) and describe myself on my social media accounts as a northern monkey, sports physio, and lover of all things aerial which basically means I spend most of my free time dangling upside down from poles, silks and hoops. I guess you could call me a 'career' woman as I spent the majority of my 20s and early 30s single, pushing myself academically and in my career, gaining a Masters degree, and travelling the world with various sports teams to the detriment of my love life. At 32 I met my now husband and gradually the time spent working decreased so we could do more together (and so I could dangle more – see above). Our relationship moved pretty quickly and within 6 months we were living together. Three years ago we moved out of my one-bedroom flat and bought our 'family' home and an SUV ready for what we hoped would come in the future.

In January 2019 Ian proposed and I quickly got around planning our wedding for February 2020. Having met later in life and spending 5 years together before getting engaged I didn't want to hang around, particularly as we both wanted children. With everything booked, a week before my hen do in November I realised I was due my period, but it didn't come. After living in denial for over a week I finally plucked up the courage to take a pregnancy test without telling my fiancé. Not because it wouldn't be welcome if it were positive, but more because of the timing – 3 months out from our wedding and 5 months out from the honeymoon of our dreams to Bora Bora. I wasn't sure how he'd react and what impact pregnancy would have on our plans. The test was positive.

Ian says he's never seen me more terrified as when I gave him the test. He was overjoyed. I had mixed emotions. I've always wanted children but the timing was terrible. My wedding dress was fitted – how would I fit in it at 4 months pregnant? Would I be ok to travel to literally the other side of the world at 5.5 months pregnant? I also have huge white coat syndrome and get terrified by doctors (ironic given my career) and knew I'd have to get over that pretty quickly. But after reassurance from Ian, my wedding dress fitter and our travel insurance I slowly got used to the idea of being pregnant. It's a weird one isn't it – as a woman you spend your whole life trying to avoid getting pregnant 'inappropriately' and then when it happens at an 'appropriate' time and in a stable relationship I still felt a bit like I had done something wrong! However, we started planning all the things you do when you find out you're expecting; which room will be the nursery, thinking about names and what sex it will be and the excitement grew.

At 7ish weeks I woke up on a Monday morning and experienced some dark brown spotting. We saw the GP, who was lovely and reassured me that she didn't think it was a sign of an ectopic pregnancy but that she would refer me to the EPAU at our local hospital for a scan. This wouldn't be for another couple of days. We told our parents, knowing that we may need their support if the news was bad. Phone calls which initially create such joy with both sets of parents, possibly about to become grandparents for the first time, but quickly create worry and desperate attempts to reassure.

Two days later, sitting in the EPAU waiting room, surrounded by other couples all with the same look of fear on their faces was tough. One by one, couples went into the ultrasound room, some came out smiling, others not. And then it was our turn. I have to give the team credit, they don't muck around and within a minute we could see our 7 week, 2 day old baby on the screen, heart beating strongly. We were one of the lucky ones who got to come out smiling. The sonographer did find I had quite a large fibroid and this was felt to be the cause of my spotting. It was such a relief.

From then on we went full gusto into pregnancy with midwife appointments, Consultant reviews (due to a possible underlying blood condition on my part) and more urine tests than anyone needs to ever do! We plotted how to tell our wider families over Christmas when I'd be just over 11 weeks and bought siblings best aunty and uncle paraphernalia to unwrap. Ginger biscuits eased my nausea and as we reached the Christmas period this started to ease and my boobs were less painful. I assumed that this was the end of the first trimester normal and in a flurry of tears and hugs families congratulated us. We went to look at prams in the sales and chose the one we wanted for our 'Little Bean'.

But on Boxing day, at our traditional rugby league match attendance, I had more spotting. It unnerved me but it was only very light and stopped quickly. The following day it came back again and was slightly heavier. I called my EPAU who suggested it was probably nothing to worry about as I didn't have pain and to wait until my 12-week scan 4 days later. I called the local EPAU in Yorkshire where we were staying with my parents later that day who again suggested waiting until my dating scan but as spotting got darker brown, I got more worried and ended up spending the night in A&E. Again I was reassured it didn't sound like a threatened miscarriage and that there were no signs of anything else and to again wait for my upcoming scan. But the following morning I knew something wasn't right with increasingly heavy dark brown spotting and so booked into the local EPAU for assessment.

My mum drove us to the hospital. I was called through pretty quickly. And this time there was no immediate reassurance. Only silence. And then after 2-3 minutes the confirmation of what I already knew. Our baby had died. And from the size, it had died pretty soon after our previous scan at 7 weeks – a 'missed' miscarriage. My mum came in. We cried. And then she left so I could undergo the internal scan needed. Now two sonographers were needed to confirm the news. And the questions - did we want to see what they could see? Did we want a photo? Was I in any pain?

And then it was over. You are no longer pregnant. You clean yourself up and cry. Midwives offer their condolences along with tea and biscuits. And then decisions. As my miscarriage was 'missed' I had to decide on how I wanted to proceed with clearing it as my body clearly wasn't doing it for me. The medication option – the least invasive but possibly most psychologically scarring, the 'vacuum' option – good if you've got a high pain threshold and can withstand the thought of your cervix being jabbed with needles and then hoovered out whilst still awake, or the traditional D&C done under anaesthetic. We were told there was at least a week's wait for a D&C and with our wedding only 4 weeks away we needed a quick 'fix'. So I opted for the medication and off we went with it and a handful of pamphlets about miscarriage and the support available.

I've only ever seen my dad cry twice – once was my wedding day and the other when I arrived home from the hospital that day. What is normally our whole family celebration day over Christmas had become a day of mourning. I had ruined Christmas and there was nothing anyone could do to help us. Ian and I spent the rest of the day sleeping and crying and cuddling, building up the courage to take the medication I knew would 'end' my pregnancy. Before I eventually took it, we spoke to the baby and took photos of our hands in the shape of a heart over my tiny bump. These are now in frames with our scan photo on our bedside windowsill so that we always remember. Not that you can forget.

They say that the medication creates symptoms of labour. Having not had children I don't know but I consider myself lucky that I only needed to take one of the 50 codeine tablets the hospital gave me to manage the pain. I bled heavily until about 3 in the morning and then I felt the baby pass. Luckily I couldn't see it in the rest of the blood but I knew from the feeling that the baby had gone. And then the pain stopped. As if nothing had happened. Just the giant sanitary towels and 3 weeks of intermittent bleeding as your constant reminder of the life that never was.

We stayed with my parents until New Years' Eve, letting them look after us. Miscarriage doesn't just affect the couple but the whole family. My parents felt useless, they couldn't ease our pain and so their way of helping was to look after us, letting us cry and being there with endless cups of tea and hugs. But they were grieving too. My mum still has days where she grieves the loss of the much-wanted grandchild that never came to be but they put their pain aside to let us wallow in ours. I don't know what we would have done without them in those first few days and that's something we'll never be able to repay.

New Year came and went and then I was due to return to work. I'd spoken to my boss shortly after my miscarriage as I was due back in work after Christmas the day after but I just wasn't sure I was ready to go back. My job involves being emotionally available to my patients and I knew I couldn't offer them that. Luckily my bosses have been incredible and I worked from home for a further week, getting my head back in the game before I saw a patient face to face. Typically my first patient back was a lady with pelvic girdle pain in pregnancy. Talk about jumping in at the deep end but I knew that wallowing in my grief any longer wasn't an option with our wedding in 3 weeks.

I have never had the guilt feelings that I know many women feel after a miscarriage. I'm not sure whether my medical background helps with the acceptance that miscarriage is 'just' something that happens, usually due to serious chromosomal abnormalities and that the child would never have survived or lived any quality of life even if they had been born. I hope that all women going through baby loss know this. It is rarely ever your fault and you should not feel any guilt. But if you do, that is also absolutely ok just please speak to someone about how you are feeling. As much as pent up grief can cause long-term mental health issues, carrying unwarranted guilt has just as profound an effect on both your mental and physical health. I have seen enough women over my career with long-term problems pain stemming back to miscarriage to validate this.

Having the wedding to focus on was certainly a useful distraction and coping tool for us in those early days. As a couple, we were also in the fortunate (?) position of having many friends to have gone through miscarriage previously, one at 20 weeks only a few months before. My coping strategy has always been to talk to my friends and have my feelings validated and supported and I think one of the most resonating things I was told in the weeks after is that miscarriage is a uniquely awful loss.

With the loss of loved ones, you have a lifetime of memories, photos, videos etc to hold onto to help cope with the loss but with a miscarriage, you have none of that, only the grief for the potential that your baby could have had and the lifetime of hopes and dreams that a baby brings. The grief is immense and it's ok to still feel that grief. A friend who lost a baby nearly 4 years ago and has gone on to have a healthy pregnancy since told me that she still lights her angel baby's candle when she feels sad about it and her family know that if that candle is lit she needs a little more TLC. My mum bought a candle for our wedding which we lit after our vows in memory of the baby. That candle now sits with the photos on our windowsill and is lit whenever I feel upset. My sister also bought me a butterfly necklace for my wedding day, the symbol of baby loss. I haven't taken it off since so our Little Bean is always with me.

It is true that time makes things easier but as I sit at my desk at work today, in the midst of the COVID-19 pandemic which thwarted our honeymoon plans, the natural 'start again' point for trying for a baby, I have realised that although time does help, for me, the quick succession of events since my miscarriage – the wedding, our 'mini-moon' to NYC, the cancellation of our 'big' honeymoon and the death of one of my best friends and that's before you stick redeployment into a new service to help with the COVID-19 response has meant that honestly I don't think I have processed my grief fully. Over the past couple of weeks I have had increasing levels of anxiety and after a lot of late-night soul searching when I should have been asleep I think it does stem back to my miscarriage. I have now admitted this to Ian and he has told me he was waiting for it all to hit again and has been incredible with his love and support, even if it has just been stroking my hair whilst I cry. Just talking to him about it has reduced some of my anxiety. I don't know whether this will be enough and have contemplated calling the Miscarriage Association at times for their help, but at the moment I'm working through it with Ian and with the help of friends and family, even if it is over Zoom! I now feel in a much better place to seriously think about trying for a baby again I know that any future pregnancy will be filled with anxieties given what happened with this one and I've had to work through the fear of even trying to get pregnant, but I'm hopeful that we will be blessed with a child sometime soon and give our Little Bean the rainbow brother or sister they deserve.

Chrissy

Chrissy and husband Greg have been trying for a baby for 10 years, and have sadly lost two babies, at 16 weeks and 19 weeks old. They continue to try for their rainbow baby.

My name is Chrissy Portnall. I'm 32 and my husband Gregory Portnall is 35 years old. We have been together for 12 years, married for 6 years on 30th May

We have been trying for a baby for 10 years. I found out I had PCOS - Polycystic Ovaries Syndrome which affects fertility in May 2013. I take 1 tablet of metformin every day to help with PCOS. Another side effect of PCOS is I have irregular periods and dark hair on the skin.

We were advised by the doctor we had to try for 2 years to conceive before they can help. After 2 years Greg and I went to doctors and it has been backwards and forwards with tests. My husband had to do 2 sperm tests and both came back low. My doctor thought it might be the case of Clomid to help me ovulate but needed to go to a fertility clinic. We went to see the consultant at Fertility Clinic in June 2014 and we were told the only option is IVF which took Greg and I by surprise as all along we were under the impression we can try Clomid. To qualify for IVF on NHS I have to lose 2 stone to be under the BMI 30 I'm currently 33 (I lost nearly 3 stone already) and my husband had stopped smoking for 6 months. As soon I walked out of the room I cried. All I wanted is to have a baby.

In April 2015 I had to force my bleed by taking Provera for 10 days and it brings on a bleed and normally it should kick in a period but unfortunately, it didn't.

Around June 2015, something made me take a pregnancy test and surprisingly it was positive. Greg and I couldn't believe it. On 4th October 2015 sadly our son George was born at 16 weeks old. I had an infection and I haemorrhaged. I lost 1 and 1/2 litre of blood. I was close to having a blood transfusion. I had to have 2 operations in space of a day due to issues with the placenta. I was in hospital for about 4 days. Greg and I were devastated, after trying for so long. Around 7 months later I fell pregnant again but sadly on 25th August 2016 Theodore was born at 19 weeks and 3 days old. I suffered with another infection which later confirmed I had sepsis. it made me seriously poorly. I was in hospital for 5 days. There were no words to describe the pain we were suffering to lose another baby within a year. When we went to see our consultant 3 months later to find out what happened, she said my cervix opened by itself and the infection hit my body, then the placenta and then inside the womb. The consultant said they will stitch my cervix up when I'm 12 weeks when I get pregnant again and that should stop my cervix to open.

A couple of months after seeing a consultant and still feeling poorly, I went to doctors, they took swabs and blood tests, and a few days later the doctor called me to say I had Strep B and I will be a carrier when I get pregnant again which I will be at high risk.

To help with our grief with spoke to a charity called SANDS that deals with miscarriage and stillbirths.

To this day we are still trying for a baby, maybe one day we will get our rainbow baby.

Instragram @chrissylouise21

Dee

Dee found strength in her husband throughout her two missed miscarriages, which lead to anxiety and depression. She continues to seek joy through kindness and her gorgeous dog Ruby and has recently found out she is pregnant again.

I am a 35 year old woman who seeks kindness, small animals and positivity as a kind of life mantra. I have an incredible husband, Alistair, who has been an integral part of my life over the last 18 years. I also have a golden dog called Ruby who brings us much joy and has been my therapy so to speak. I love my job in Learning & Development, helping people to reflect, become self-aware and hopefully be more effective managers. I haven't always wanted babies - I'll put that out there now. It took A and I a long time to get to the place of deciding to try. Lots of our doubt was whether we could do it. I've felt emotionally all over the place for a long time and have grappled with an eating disorder (in secret) for most of my adult life. I was really good at looking like I had my shit together, like I was making the most of everything - super busy at work, volunteering in my spare time, trying lots of new hobbies and wanting to be everything to everyone.

My story is that I've had two missed miscarriages. I didn't know that much about miscarriages before we got pregnant, let alone what a missed miscarriage was. We had some close friends who lost babies, in both first and second trimesters and we saw the absolute devastation it caused. This still didn't prepare us for the storm of emotions that was to come.

In our first pregnancy, we were a couple of days away from our 12 week scan when I had some brown discharge. I spent all day in a state of anxiety before I called the early pregnancy unit (EPU) to see what I needed to do. They advised coming in for a scan the following day. We found out on 3rd Dec 2018 that our baby had died and had surgical management on 6th Dec. I was absolutely broken, we really thought we would be ok. That we would have a baby. That pregnancy = a baby. I had a bit of time off work after the surgery and then tried to go back. It was too hard and I took 4 weeks off work in the early part of 2019.

Life slowly got a bit better, we found some joy again and even though we were trying, part of me was terrified of getting pregnant again. I felt raw and exposed from dealing with my eating disorder too and finally recognising that my mental health was not in a great place.

A and I signed up to do the Ride London event in August 2019 and it felt good to have a focus. We went out for 40 miles each weekend and went to spin classes 2-3 times a week so exercise helped us to stay strong. That sounds like we're highly motivated gym-goers - don't get the wrong impression! Our motivation came in peaks and troughs and the pressure of the ride was constantly there for us - so really, I'm not sure it did help that much other than to get us exercising.

In June 2019, we found out we were pregnant for the second time. I sobbed when I saw the test was positive. How could it be? How could I do it? How could we do it? The anxiety was super high from the outset and looking back now, I wasn't emotionally ready for it. We tried to connect with the pregnancy the best we could and had some lovely adventures in the early weekend, such a weekend away in Copenhagen for A's birthday where we did a long bike ride too. The week following this trip, I was at work about to start a coaching workshop when I had the tiniest bit of blood on some tissue after going to the loo. The panic was instant and I honestly don't know how I got through that day.

We managed to get a scan for the following day and it was inconclusive - we were measuring a week behind and they couldn't detect a heartbeat however they said that was fairly normal and to come back in 10 days. I dipped between hope and despair during those 10 days and again, I don't know how I got through them. I sobbed most days at the possibility of losing our baby again.

10 days later and our fears were confirmed - the baby hadn't grown at all and there was still no heartbeat. I was booked in for surgery a week later - another period of waiting - either to bleed naturally or to go in for that same operation.

The waiting during all of the above contributed to my decline in mental health - my anxiety has never been worse than it was around this missed miscarriage. A couple of days after the surgery (I didn't bleed naturally - one of the biggest challenges I've found with losing two babies is the lack of trust in my own body - when I already had such deep-rooted issues going on) I had my first panic attack and it scared me so much. I spent days with my heart racing and feeling like my throat was closed up. I couldn't get enough oxygen. I was a mess.

I went back to work 2 weeks after the surgery and managed a month at work before I truly recognised that I was not doing well. I was depressed and my anxiety was gripping me tightly. I was just about getting through my days at work with the odd session of breathing somewhere quiet to stop my heart from pounding or sitting in my car crying as I was too overwhelmed.

I was signed off work with anxiety and depression and started taking medication. This was a HUGE deal for me. I am such a supporter of people doing what they need to look after themselves, meds and all. But for myself - it felt like I'd failed. I'd been working hard in counselling for over a year on and off and this had helped me tremendously. I was sure I was supposed to be dealing with it by myself and continue life with this broken part of myself. But anti-depressants. In my body. What about if we wanted to get pregnant again? Surely that would not be good for the baby? What if they made me into a zombie? What if all of this meant I couldn't cope with life?

Well - I wasn't coping with anything and it took me several weeks to allow my mind to settle into helping myself get better. The meds only helped once the dose was increased and then I felt glimmers of hope again. I was off work for a couple of months. I borrowed a dog to help - he was the best type of therapy. I had acupuncture and reflexology. I took long walks every day. I slept a lot. I watched A LOT of Grey's Anatomy. I baked. I cried. I meditated. I did nothing some days. In the midst of all of this, I definitely felt suicidal. I never admitted that to the GP when she asked me. Or my therapist. I talked about it with A once I was out of the worst of it, several months on and I realised how real that plan was for me. I'm so very glad now that I did not try to end my life. I think I had my Samaritans volunteer training in the back of my mind too and knowing so much about suicide and the impact was always there for me.

It took 6 months for my period to return following the second loss - I am truly thankful for my body doing what it needed to do and protecting me. At the time, I was frustrated, of course.

I wouldn't have been able to get to where I am now without such incredible support from those close to me - Alistair is just incredible and has his own story and experience of our loss and he supported me - he held me most days as I sobbed deeply into his chest. Such painful crying and he was and is amazing.

Instagram: deannelogan2017

Ellie

*Ellie has grappled with many a 'what if?' and feelings of guilt
throughout her journey, but a particular book is helping her find a new
way of approaching a future possibly without children. She feels
strongly about the perception of motherhood in society.*

My name is Ellie, I'm 36 years old. I used to be an
actress and I lived in London for 8 years where I met my
partner. For the last 5 years I have worked in Human
Resources and in 2017 my partner and I moved up to
Warwick in the Midlands.

I had always known that I wanted to be a mother,
there was never a doubt in my mind. In fact, I had long ago
come to the conclusion that it was what I wanted most in
life. Whenever I faced something tough to deal with or
failed at something, it was my compensation thought – "it's
okay, one day I will be a mother, and that will make up for
this difficult time; going through this shitty thing now is
how I earn the privilege of being a mother later in life; so I
failed at this, that's okay, because I'll be an excellent
mother one day and that will be my purpose in life...". I had
always assumed that I would be a mother, that it was my
destiny, as it was for so many women. I debated whether I
would have 3 or 4 children, I stored my old toys in my
parents' loft assuming I would pass them on to my children
one day, I held on to pictures that would look great in a

nursery, I added baby names to a list saved on my phone, and I would casually say things to my partner like "we'll come here with the kids one day", "the kids won't believe it when I tell them we did this one day" etc.

But looking back, I also see that I also carried a small but real anxiety deep inside me, that I would perhaps be one of those women (like my Aunt) who would never get the chance to conceive or raise a child. A paranoia that I would be the unlucky one. I carried this small yet hefty anxiety around with me because essentially it was my biggest fear in life, a nightmare scenario which I hoped and reassured myself was unlikely. Even so, knowing that women's fertility decreases rapidly after 30 I spent my twenties earnestly seeking a life partner.

At the start of 2014, a month after my 30th birthday, I finally found him - Mike. On our first date, much to my friend's horror, I asked whether he saw himself being a father one day. This is how important parenthood was to me. We fell in love quickly and we are still very much in love today. He is my rock, exceptionally wonderful and I feel so lucky to call him my husband. We often joke about how we wished we had found each other sooner. We married just under three years after meeting one another in December 2016. Impressive, considering I spent a good 6 months of our courtship very poorly indeed. Three months after we married, having not long turned 33, we started trying for a child.

Three years later at the age of 36, we are still trying. Unexplained Infertility – the phrase is a metaphorical shrug of the shoulders, and it sucks. It leaves you with so many unanswered questions and "what-ifs". Anatomically there is no reason why we should not have conceived by now.

I was diagnosed with Crohn's Disease in 2014, a condition in which parts of the digestive system become inflamed and ulcerated, and in early 2015, a year into my new relationship with Mike, I suffered a severe flare-up. I was hospitalised for three months, and had my large intestine completely removed and a stoma constructed. The medics tell me that there appears to be no damage caused by the abdominal surgery that would affect my fertility, but of course I am left questioning if this is the case. I also wonder whether purely having a chronic underlying illness makes my body reject pregnancy, deciding it won't be able to carry a baby full term, despite me knowing that other women with Crohn's and stomas have successfully conceived, carried and given birth to children.

I do have an unexplained and shockingly low egg count for my age (more akin to that of the average 48 year old) but in theory this shouldn't have affected my ability to conceive naturally over the last 3 years either, as the quality of the eggs I release each month should be the same as any other 30-something women. It does however mean that I probably have less time to make this baby thing happen! Is my low egg reserve due to my underlying health condition, the result of the powerful medications I had to take whilst ill, or the excessive mental stress of the hospital stay? More unanswered questions.

I also seem to be prone to polyps (which are essentially like skin tags that grow inside your womb), but again, these should not necessarily have a big impact on my ability to conceive or carry a child. I'm told women with polyps often conceive, carry and give birth without even knowing they have them. My polyps were discovered mid-way through my first and only NHS-funded IVF cycle. My only suitable egg from this cycle was therefore frozen and only transferred back into my womb once I had undergone a procedure to remove the polyps a few months later. The IVF cycle failed. Another "what-if" to deal with... "what if the medics had discovered the polyp before IVF... would the egg have had a better chance if it was fresh rather than frozen?" And perhaps some anger that they didn't spot the polyp sooner too.

Fertility treatment is a rollercoaster of emotions. I would often feel guilty about something – "If I had avoided catching a cold after the egg was transferred, the IVF cycle may have been successful". You often feel like you should be doing more of something or less of something. More yoga, more acupuncture, more vitamins, more positive thinking. Get a less stressful job, think less about conceiving, ride your bike less. But let's get real, people with bad health or unhealthy lifestyles conceive, people exposed to horrendous emotional, mental and physical turmoil conceive. No amount of willing-it, not-thinking-about-it, Pilates, bed rest, meditation, or vitamins (unless you have a genuine deficiency) is likely to make a difference if your body just doesn't want you to conceive. Your infertility is not because you are or aren't doing something, it's not your fault, it's just nature being a bitch. When someone tells you "My friend has been trying for years, started reflexology and got pregnant in days!" politely thank this person for their advice but let them know that it was almost certainly a coincidence and that there were probably another 10 women who tried reflexology and are still childless. When you're told "You're trying too hard or thinking too much about it", politely ask them to show you where they found the 'off' button on their mind and also ask them to show you the research study that confirms this theory! You really must not blame yourself or let others make you feel responsible for your own infertility, something which is completely out of your control. I know their advice is well-meaning, but they really need to get a medical degree before they dish out their guidance.

After our failed NHS funded IVF attempt, we tried NHS funded intrauterine insemination and ovarian stimulation drugs for 6 months with no success. So in early 2020, now feeling guilty (there's that word again) that we hadn't come to this decision sooner, we decided we would fund our own round of IVF. But fate was once again not on our side. A new small polyp had grown in my womb. Ideally, it needed removing before we could undertake IVF to give ourselves the best chance of a successful pregnancy. So three years after we started this journey, our self-funded attempt was being pushed back by a further 2 months to undergo the polypectomy. Of course, the procedure scheduled for April 2nd 2020 never went ahead, as COVID-19 saw to that. At the time of writing in early June 2020, I am still awaiting my 'routine procedure', having had it cancelled three times due to the Coronavirus outbreak. Given that my low egg count means time is of the essence, with every month passing potentially making the difference between becoming parents or not, you can imagine how upsetting and frustrating this is for us. It feels like the sands of hope are rapidly escaping through our fingertips.

Even if we manage to undergo IVF before I completely run out of eggs, my low egg count makes achieving a successful round of IVF more difficult. Even with the stimulating drugs, I am likely to produce fewer eggs (or potentially no eggs) which in turn reduces the chances of the cycle ending with a fertilised egg ready for transfer.

So after 3 years and 2 months of 'trying', we find ourselves facing the prospect that our fertility story might not have a happy ending. Cue more guilt – "are we childless because I'm being punished for being a dickhead sometimes; is this punishment for not believing in God?", and self-directed anger – "we should have sought medical advice sooner; we should have pursued self-funded IVF more aggressively at the start; we should have started trying before we got married." Even if you can get past blaming yourself, you are left with an immense feeling of injustice. Why me?! Of all the people for this to happen to, why did it have to be me, the person who so resolutely wanted children for so long. The person who would have made a wonderful mother, the person who had made sensible life choices and sacrifices to ensure a stable and loving home for her future family. Coming to terms with the fact that life just isn't fair is still something I'm struggling with. It makes me intensely angry. I felt like I had built a belief system on equity and fairness and now I find myself living in a world I don't recognise and don't like because it isn't fair. If life isn't fair, what's the point in participating in it or being a good person? It feels like you've been playing a board game and halfway through someone suddenly changes the rules. You want to tip the board over, shout "I don't want to play anymore" and run to your room in a strop. Of course, I realise now that the injustice I felt reveals an ugly side of me. I had built a belief system not on equity and fairness but on entitlement and superiority. I don't doubt that many women feel an entitlement to become a mother – and that is why it's so hard when we learn we cannot be one – but it's not right to believe that I am more deserving of having a child than any other women. What a shameful thing to believe! The stable home I built did involve some sacrifices, but being in a position to make those sacrifices indicates how I was already in a position of privilege. Confronting this ugly and bitter side of myself whilst dealing with my infertility is difficult. It's another weapon to torment myself with. I must acknowledge it, learn from it, but not allow myself to conclude my misgivings are why fate decided to not make me a mother. Life's setbacks, such as infertility, are perhaps more difficult to comprehend and accept if you have led a life of privilege. Whilst I have had to deal with poor health and learn to accept that my dream career was not to be, in truth, prior to my late twenties, I led a pretty idyllic life.

This did not prepare me well to deal with disappointments – they are something I am simply not used to experiencing. I have not developed the coping mechanisms and resilience to deal with them. "Why me?" I asked myself, well, why not me?! Bad things happen, get used to it like others have had to...

I'm currently in a limbo, all at once clasping onto the last sands of hope that if our self-funded IVF cycle ever goes ahead, that it might, against all odds, actually work, whilst simultaneously feeling immense feelings of anger and sadness as I realise I will likely never conceive, carry or give birth to a child. Within one day I can be found ignoring friends calls to isolate away from the cruel world I no longer want to participate in, becoming incredibly angry when others, in my opinion, behave immorally or unfairly, saying cruel and downright nasty things to provoke reactions from others or make them hurt as I do, uncontrollably crying into my pillow with pity that I will never cradle a baby in my arms, and casually starting a sentence "when we have kids...." Not an easy way to live your life.

Before you say "well, she could adopt", let me say this. Adoption, in my opinion, is probably a far more complex and emotionally gruelling experience than fertility treatment could ever be - and only once you have either done it or genuinely looked into doing it and making it your reality, can you begin to understand the complexities and emotions involved. Please do not think you are qualified to judge whether another person could or should do it. I marvel at those who do choose to do it, who have the strength of character to weather its ups and downs. And whilst it is something we are considering very seriously, I am also acutely aware that having been physically and emotionally abused by our fertility journey over the last three years, that we may not yet be, or ever be, emotionally or mentally resilient enough to undertake this route to parenthood. And if we aren't able to, and if all our IVF treatments fail, how do we come to terms with a future that is not the one we so wanted and expected. A future I couldn't even imagine being happy living? A childless future!

I have found myself seeking help from the childless community, as this could be how my story ends - or starts, depending on your point of view...

I would wholeheartedly recommend that anyone facing a childless future, for whatever reason, joins the Gateway Women Community set up by Jody Day. I am currently reading her book "Living the Life Unexpected" and am astounded at how articulately she manages to capture so many of my feelings and thoughts. Realising that there are other women out there with shared experiences you can talk to is so very comforting. In truth, I feel everyone should read her book, so others can gain some understanding of what it's like to be a childless woman in today's society and better see how society as a whole is doing women a disservice in the way we view motherhood and childlessness.

Jody Day made me realise that I must allow myself to mourn the loss of the children I will not have. They are as real to me as any other women's born children. I pictured bringing them home from the maternity ward, taking a photo of them on their first day of school, disapproving of their first boyfriend, celebrating with them when they pass their driving test, proudly attending their wedding and even being a grandparent to their children one day. I appreciate of course, that if I had had children, this idealised vision of what it would have been like would be nothing like the reality, but their souls and my bond to them are still real. I love them, despite the fact that they were never born, and I must therefore grieve that they have been taken from me. Furthermore, others must allow me to do this and respect that I need to.

I'm also learning that I should not feel guilty about the way I react to certain situations, such as friends announcing pregnancies or seeing young families out enjoying themselves. Jody Day has taught me to treat them as opportunities to further my healing as part of the grieving process. I want to release myself from the negative power they have over me. This is something I am still working on.

The thought of a childless existence was my worst nightmare, and whilst I still desperately desire to be a mother one day, should I never be one, the childless community has made me realise that I will go on living, I will have moments of joy in my life and live a fulfilling existence, growing around my grief as others do when they lose family members. Looking back, I cringe at the thought that I ever wanted to be defined by motherhood alone, that I was happy to consider this as being my only purpose in life. A friend of mine recently became pregnant and instantly changed her Instagram bio to read 'Mother-to-be' and changed her picture to display her bump. I was shocked. This woman is a very intelligent and accomplished individual, with a myriad of facets that define who she is. To reduce herself to a baby-producing and -rearing entity seemed inexplicably wrong to me. Jody Day's book has been truly enlightening in regards to its analysis of how our society views and treats both mothers and childless women, how most of us unwittingly feed into this narrative, and how damaging this ideology is to both. It's a complex issue and one I cannot begin to summarise here, but it is clear to me now that placing mothers on a pedestal and upholding the notion that raising children is the key to a woman's happiness and fulfilment is unhelpful and damaging for all women. Despite what we are encouraged to believe, a mother is no more valuable to society than a childless woman. Childless women have been marginalised by our society. Despite childlessness being the fate of a large number of women these days, it is something never discussed, so taboo that even those it happens to rarely discuss it between them. Having to come to terms with being childless not by choice is up there as one of the most heart-breaking ordeals you could imagine having to deal with, yet it is one for which there is very little support or empathy, and very little public discourse about. These women who are in need of support while they grieve find themselves more isolated than most. When a woman facing a childless future starts to tell you how upsetting it is and you respond with messages of positivity, saying that she shouldn't give up hope or that you know someone who got pregnant who thought they couldn't, you are effectively silencing them. You are saying, I don't want to hear your sad story because it makes me feel uncomfortable, please be positive for my sake so that I don't have to imagine what it would be like if I personally had to go through what you are having to go through. This is why we hear a disproportionate number of fertility stories with happy endings, despite 75% of fertility treatment ending in failure. This is why I was so keen to take part in this project. To give a voice to those whose stories make us feel uncomfortable.

Along with the childless community, I have also received a great deal of support from my family and friends. I feel so lucky that I have felt comfortable to share with them the details of our journey and my thoughts and feelings, and that they, in turn, have been so understanding and supportive. I know not all women are fortunate in this way, but I would encourage you to open up to others, and where you receive the support you need, continue to seek it there. Where you do not, accept that not everyone has the emotional maturity to respond appropriately and don't waste your energy trying to get them to. Talking honestly and openly about fertility, motherhood and childlessness is key to reducing stigmas associated with these subjects. Everyone's story is important, not just those that have a happy ending.

It goes without saying that my husband's support and love has been unfaltering and we both realise more and more each day how lucky we are to have one another.

Finally, I would recommend seeking counselling through your fertility clinic which is available on the NHS. Even if you only attend a couple of sessions, I think it's important to give time and space to discuss how the journey is affecting you and your relationships.

I hope this letter helps someone in some way.

Emily

Meet Emily, who felt that she wasn't taken seriously in regard to her periods as a teen and young adult, which affected her trust in doctors further down the line. This is also reflected in her brief account of birth partway through her story.

Let me begin by saying that I am aware my story is very mild compared to the challenges and heartbreak many women experience. I count myself very fortunate when I hear some of the traumas my friends have gone through; losing multiple babies, and in a few cases nearly their own lives. My experiences don't compare on this level, nonetheless if my sharing can help anyone in any way I am more than happy to do so, and I actually found it to be quite cathartic for myself through putting it all to paper.

Periods:
My Periods were genuinely the bane of my life! I wasn't worried about my period starting as a child as in all the sex-education classes we'd been reassured that the first few times they would be light and painless – all lies! My period started when I was 11 years old in the summer between primary school and secondary school. I'd been singing as part of a choir at a nice couple's wedding and started to feel unwell – tummy cramps and nausea, and presumed I was getting an upset tummy. I walked the 10-

minute journey home which felt like forever and went straight to the loo, and there was all the blood! It was a shock, and I did scream a little (but then I was only 11!), I then spent the next 2 hours rolling around the floor in agony with increasing stomach cramps, which caused me to vomit, have diarrhea, and nearly pass out on several occasions. Thankfully my mother was a midwife of 20+ years' experience, and dealt with it all calmly and patiently. Thus began the next 5 years of hell...

These periods, which only got worse in pain, and heavier each month (usually lasting 10+ days) left me exhausted and anaemic, and caused me to miss at least 2 days of school per month (depending on which days of the week they fell on) due to the pain. My school work was affected, as was my confidence, as I was one of the first girls in my class to have periods and I didn't feel able to talk to any of my friends about it. My periods were also extremely heavy and I would often have leaks during class and have to go to the toilet frequently.

My parents took me to the doctor on numerous occasions, and each time was told 'these things are normal', 'it's just period pain', 'give her some pain relief', 'they'll settle as she gets older', or my personal favourite 'they'll sort themselves out once she has a baby'... I was 11 years old at this point! My Dad, bless him, (who I was mortified even knew I had periods) found an interesting article when I was about 12 years old on Endometriosis which he took to the doctors, but they pretty much laughed us out of the surgery, it was so embarrassing.

When I was 14 my period came on at school during a PE lesson, and I went to the toilet and passed out and vomited all over the bathroom floor. Thankfully someone found me and went to get the teacher. My PE teacher (a brisk abrupt lady) came in and tried to put her jumper under my head whilst I lay on the floor, and apparently I vomited all over it! An ambulance was called and to my humiliation, I was carted out in front of the school during lunchtime and taken off to hospital.

At hospital the first thing they asked (in front of the aforementioned teacher) was 'are you pregnant?', as these pains couldn't just be simply period pains. I was so embarrassed and upset and confirmed that no I couldn't be pregnant. A few minutes later my teacher went to get a drink, and again the nurses came in and strongly pressed me as to whether I was pregnant or not. I know they have to ask, but once again it just felt like another medical person not listening to me trying to explain how bad the pain really was.

After this, I was given some tablets to help manage my periods called Mefenamic Acid. I tried to take these as directed 3x per day the 3 days leading up to my period, but my periods weren't always regular. Sometimes I would forget to take them to school (being a forgetful teenage girl), and these pills had the nasty side effect of giving me excruciating back pain within 30 mins of taking them (I could almost set a timer to it). Again I went to the doctors to discuss this pain and they said they'd never heard of it happening before (i.e. you're either making it up, or just a confused little girl).

Finally, when I was 15 years old my Mum took me to the doctors to ask if I could go on the combined Pill. It was a Godsend! For the next 4 years, my periods went from 10+ to 7 days in length, became much more regular, and while the pain was still bad and required continual paracetamol, ibuprofen, hot water bottle, and me to not move for the day, it wasn't the vomit and diarrhoea-inducing hell I'd had for the previous 4 years.

When I was 18 years old I was diagnosed with hypothyroidism (an underactive thyroid) and put on life-long daily medication to manage, and was told this may also help to settle my periods down as it can have an adverse effect when not functioning properly.

Things were good until I was 19 years old. I'd always had hormone-induced migraines (lasting 1 day a month around the week of my period), but when I was a university these migraines became more intense and frequent (1 or 2 a week), until they got so bad that I had one that lasted 5 days, the side of my face went completely numb, and I couldn't get out of bed; thankfully my very new boyfriend was super and made sure I was alright and tried to get me to eat something each day. My boyfriend wisely insisted I go to the doctors, so once I could get out of bed I went and as I had feared they said it was highly likely that the Pill was causing these migraines, and as they were migraines with auras (I didn't have the flashing lights, but my face going numb was a type of aura) I had to come off them immediately as I was at risk of having a stroke. I was not happy about this, obviously I wasn't going to risk a stroke, however the memory of how awful these periods had been still stuck with me, which I tried to explain to the doctor. After making the same old, frequently heard quip about how they would settle down if I had a baby... (again I was 20 years old at this point and at Uni, so a baby was not on my to-do list), the doctor felt I should try a few months without anything to give my body a break, and see how bad my periods were now I was older; if that didn't work I could try different types of contraception to see what worked.

I won't bore you with the details, but basically while my periods were ok at first, they gradually got heavier and more painful over the next 6 months to the point where they became unmanageable again (thankfully my aforementioned boyfriend was super supportive, looking after me and getting me painkillers, hot water bottles, and picking me up off the floor each month). So off I headed back to the doctors and was put on the mini pill for several months. Unfortunately, this pill caused weekly breakthrough bleeding; I then had the injection – which worked for a couple of weeks, but then led to the same breakthrough bleeding, and my hormones were all over the place. I was then offered the implant, but as this was the same hormones as the mini-pill and injection I declined (as once it was put in it wasn't so easy to just remove at the drop of a hat). The doctor also suggested trying the coil, but I didn't like the idea of a foreign object sat there in my uterus. For some reason, I decided I would once again persevere with nothing and give my body a break from all these hormones.

Similarly to last time, for the first couple of months all seemed well, and I got my hopes up, but once again they began to get gradually worse – heavier, and more painful. I was determined to persevere (stubbornness on my part), until one day when I was standing at the Post Office I passed out due to the pain in front of everyone. The staff offered to call an ambulance but I declined as I was so embarrassed and knew I just needed to get home to bed. I managed to get home and took (perhaps a little too many ibuprofen), but it did the trick, and within 2 hours the pain was manageable again.

The following month I was alone in my flat and the pain came on so suddenly and severely I didn't know what to do and was worried about passing out when no one was there to keep an eye on me. I panicked and called an ambulance. They took me to A&E where a nurse angrily asked me if I often called ambulances for tummy aches. I admit it was an overreaction, but these pains were not just 'tummy aches, they were no longer manageable, I had been scared and I hadn't known what else to do. They gave me various pain relief but as nothing helped they admitted me to the ward where they administered a strong pain relief by suppository (I was so embarrassed after, but at the time I was in so much pain I didn't really care), and the relief within a couple of minutes was wonderful. I again asked about what could be causing the pain to be bad, and whether it could be Endometriosis, but they said it was unlikely and I was released the next day and told to go to the doctors to discuss options.

As I was planning my wedding at the time I spoke to the doctor about whether I could go on a different type of the combined Pill temporarily to manage my periods over my wedding and honeymoon period and the doctor agreed, but said if I had migraines again I would need to come straight back. At 23 I got married, went on honeymoon, and all was ok for a good while (no migraines and manageable periods). We moved house (which meant I changed doctors), and I settled into a new job, but slowly the migraines came back. I waited longer than I maybe should have again, but finally relented and went to the doctors (leading to the lengthy explanations about my periods, how they weren't manageable off the pill, but the pill was causing migraines, no I couldn't try the mini-pill as this didn't work, no regular painkillers didn't manage it, no I didn't want to have a baby to settle everything down, no I wasn't being pathetic and unable to manage basic tummy-aches etc. etc.) Thankfully after I practically had a meltdown in the doctor's office he agreed to refer me to see a Gynaecologist.

The Gynaecologist was nice, and listened, got me to keep a period diary over the next 4 months, and sent me for a scan to see if I had Endometriosis. The scan came back inconclusive, as they said if I had small amounts they might not show up on a scan, and there could be different amounts present at different times of the month (while obviously I didn't want anything to be 'wrong' I had hoped they might find something they could fix). The Gynaecologist said she could send me for a laparoscopy (a small procedure where they put a camera inside through an incision near the belly-button), but she would prefer to explore other avenues first. I mentioned there had been one painkiller (in suppository form at the hospital) which had helped and thankfully she agreed to prescribe me more of these, she also did a blood test to check my iron levels and found that while my iron levels were borderline, my iron stores were very low (likely due to the lengthily heavy periods) and so also prescribed me daily iron tablets. Overall I was so relieved with this appointment, the only interesting thing to note was when I received a copy of the letter she wrote to my doctor updating him on the situation, and it made reference to my being an intelligent woman, with a university degree... it just made me wonder whether they wouldn't have taken me as seriously if I hadn't proven on paper to have a couple of brain cells!?

When I was 27 my husband and I moved again, and this meant once again changing doctors. This time the doctor called me in as they wanted to ask me why I was on these strong suppositories. This led to once again my trying to explain everything about my periods, them asking if I'd tried taking paracetamol or ibuprofen before...(seriously!) and them basically asking if I was just not able to handle simple period pains. Thankfully I passed their interrogation, and they agreed to carry on prescribing the painkillers to me.

During these years off the pill, my husband and I were only able to use a limited amount of contraception, and we'd had a couple of pregnancy scares. Please don't get me wrong, we were married and if we'd gotten pregnant it wouldn't have been a bad thing as we wanted to have a family, however we weren't ready just yet; I know no one ever really is 'ready', but we wanted to have a bit more savings in the bank first, and feel more prepared. So I spoke to the doctor about what options I had, and they suggested going on the Mirena Coil. So when I was 29 years old I had the coil fitted. I know some people think it's wonderful, but personally for me it was a big mistake and I wouldn't recommend it to anyone! I had a 6 month long period and was a hormonal wreck. I had what I could only describe as PMS almost every day. But I was reassured that these symptoms would settle, and on the one hand, it worked wonders as a contraceptive(!) The periods did finally settle down, but the hormones didn't, and I put on a lot of weight. I was trying to undertake my second master's degree, and it was having an impact on this too, so I decided I needed to come off it so I went to the clinic to ask for it to be removed. Crazily as they only had one member of staff who was qualified to remove it, due to their workload it took 3 trips to this clinic over the space of a month (as they only saw non-urgent patients once a week), and several hours of sitting in the waiting room before they were available to take it out. It may sound silly, but it was an awful month, there was this foreign object in my body, making me a hormonal crazy person, and I was completely at the mercy of this one individual as to whether it would be removed or not. Finally it was removed and my body did not react well. I had crazily heavy and irregular periods, and had to go to the doctors again. They once again referred me for a scan to see if they could figure out what was going on, and again the scans came back inconclusive, but they offered to do a laparoscopy to get a more detailed picture. By this time I was in my 30s and decided, 'screw it'; I've been told all my life that having a baby will fix my periods, why don't we just start trying. So I declined the laparoscopy and was told if I wasn't pregnant in a year to come back and see them for further tests.

Conception:
We knew it could take a while to get pregnant, especially with my thyroid condition, and if I did have endometriosis, so we tried in a relaxed manner for 3 months, and unsurprisingly had no luck. So we then tried a more methodical approach, and to our joy, we became pregnant after a further 3 months. I am very appreciative of this, having seen many friends trying for years either with no luck, or joy following years of painful IVF treatments or hormone therapies, either to be lucky, or to once again experience the heartbreak of repeated miscarriages. My pregnancy went ok-ish, we had a scare at 6 weeks when I experienced bad stomach pains and a heavy bleed, we had to wait 2 days for a scan and were convinced we had lost the baby (it was an emotional and physically painful few days), but amazingly we went for the scan and to our shock and joy found out our baby was still there, its little heart beating away!

My thyroid levels and iron levels went completely off-kilter during my pregnancy, which led to me looking like a pincushion with the amount of blood tests I had, and I had to follow the high-risk consultant route (my hopes for a relaxed home birth going out the window). We also had a scare when my brother was rushed to hospital and put in the high dependency unit with a burst artery (with no apparent cause). He had to undergo many investigations and tests for various genetic disorders including Ehlers-Danlos Syndrome, which resulted in my having to go for various tests, heart scans, and be closely monitored as several possibilities could have had life-threatening implications for myself and/or baby. In this respect I cannot fault the Health professionals, as being pregnant I was seen as a priority (in fact I felt a little guilty about this as I saw some specialists while my brother, who had almost died, sat on their waiting list!), and saw a specialist and was diagnosed with a benign form of EDS (my brother still has no conclusive answers).

After birth:

I know it's not the main focus here, but I feel a little note on birth and after birth is warranted – I, having a midwife for a mother, felt very prepared for birth and like most people, had seen shows such as 'one born every minute'. What I was not prepared for, and something such shows don't focus on is what happens after you've given birth.

My little boy did not want to arrive, so due to a number of factors – my getting labyrinthitis a week before he was due, my baby measuring small, and then his weight plateauing, it was decided we would go for an induction at 41+2 weeks. I had my waters broken at 6pm, and then as nothing was happening I was put on the drip to try to get things going quickly, and boy did they! A few minutes after the midwife left the room to check on other patients, and my husband left to get a sandwich the contractions started. They didn't start slowly and gradually increase as I'd expected, they hit with full force, I felt the need to push immediately, and they stayed that intense for the next 2.5hr hours until to the surprise of the midwives my baby arrived!!

Due to the speed at which my little boy arrived, I had multiple internal and external tears and bleeds, and required a lot of stitching up, and I feel this is one of the key things we as women are not prepared for – the weeks and weeks of pain and bleeding that follow our miracle baby's arrival! Suddenly you're presented with this baby, you have no idea what to do, you're exhausted, trying to feed them from increasingly sore, swollen and bleeding nipples, all whilst you can't even sit down from the pain of all the tears and stitched in your undercarriage! In fact, the midwife actually had to remove a couple of the stitches early as they had, shall we say, sewn me up a little too far... and created knots of skin that I was told would likely need 'addressing' once I was healed.

At the 6 week check when the doctor is meant to check both you and the baby I had a male doctor who checked my son, but didn't check me (not physically to see how I was healing up, or emotionally to see how I was coping as a new parent and for any signs of postnatal depression – which looking back now I know I definitely had, at least mildly). I asked if he needed to check me and he said no. After 8 weeks the bleeding stopped, but the swelling and pain remained long after. On numerous occasions my husband and I tried to resume our sex life, but the pain was so bad we had to stop (thankfully my husband, who was the same previously mentioned amazingly supportive boyfriend, is one of the most caring and supportive men I have ever known and never made me feel embarrassed or like I was letting him down at any point, even though I felt these things myself). After 8 months of things still not working properly, I went back to the doctors – I should have gone sooner, but after all the humiliating trips where I felt I wasn't being taken seriously with my periods I don't really like going to the doctors. Thankfully the doctor agreed that things weren't as they should be and sent me to see a gynaecologist.

The Gynaecologist was not particularly sympathetic. He explained, after a very painful examination that I had a lot of scar tissue and knotted skin both internally and externally. They could operate, but as I wanted to have another baby at some point I was likely to just tear again and this would result in even more scarring, he basically said (and apologies for the oversharing) that the skin wasn't stretching as it should and that I and my husband would have to gradually stretch it out (and they say you can still maintain romance after having a baby...!). Thankfully my wonderful husband was again super supportive and with his help and understanding over the next 6 months we gradually resumed normal marital life.

Fertility:

My husband and I had decided early on that we'd like our children to be close in age, obviously the fact we couldn't really have sex properly for the first year after my son was born slowed this process down, but once we felt able to we decided to start trying for another baby. Naively we thought that after having conceived reasonably quickly the first time, things would be the same this time around, so we weren't really prepared when 6 months came and went and there was no baby. We went and bought the home fertility testing kits and for the next 6 months we were on a mission, but sadly the year mark came and went, and still no baby. I know a year is the norm, but when you have to each month not only see a negative pregnancy result, but then deal with ever increasing period pains again it is disheartening. I will give the doctors credit, while the pains are still bad, having a baby did settle my periods down from the previous 7-10 days to a much more reasonable 5-7 days, and I haven't passed out with the pain yet...!

I went to the doctors at the year mark, I know it was still reasonably early in our trying, but my concern was that whilst these were only home kits, many months I wasn't getting a positive ovulation test, even though I had begun testing on every day of the month, not just the recommended days 10-19 (cycle depending). The doctor said to carry on trying and come back in another 6 months if we still hadn't conceived. So we carried on, and we had a couple of months where my period was really late (one lasting 39 days) and we got our hopes up, but still no baby.

Again I know we were still in the very early days but I found it emotional, and my heart goes out even more to all my friends who had been trying for years. I can't imagine the emotional toll this has taken on them as an individual and also as a couple! During this time I was also made redundant and had to start a new job, which I know wouldn't have helped with my stress levels, which can impact on fertility.

By 15 months my husband and I decided the regimented approach wasn't working as we were getting too stressed about it, and tried to relax things and go back to having sex when we actually wanted to (and on the more likely days). Our hope of having our babies close in age was fading fast, but I know these things can't be planned. At the 18 month mark I booked myself an appointment at the doctors, my appointment was on the Wednesday, but my period wasn't due until the Friday, so to be sure I wasn't pregnant that month (I knew it was unlikely but I didn't want to waste the doctors time) I bought a pack of 3 expensive early detection tests, which allow you to test as early as 5 days before you are due. So I used one each day on days 26, 27 and 28 of my cycle, and unsurprisingly they all came back negative (I had also done this as I had a dentist appointment and required some x-rays and didn't want to risk having them if I was pregnant). So I went along to the doctors and as we had been trying for 18+ months the doctor agreed to refer me to a Fertility Clinic, which I was very grateful to her for.

By the Sunday my period still hadn't arrived, and while I didn't think I was pregnant I was bored and found an old cheap pregnancy test at the back of a cupboard and did it just as something to do... and to my absolute shock 2 little lines appeared!!!!! I didn't want to get my hopes up as it seemed so ridiculous that the expensive tests had all come back negative, and this tiny cheap test was now saying positive, so later that day we drove to the shop and I bought a couple of tests, and for the next 2 days I took one each morning and they all came back as positive!

I can't express the joy and relief I felt, but also the fear of something bad happening (especially as I'd had those dental x-rays). While I was aware of all the things that could go wrong in pregnancy with my first baby, because we hadn't had any trouble conceiving we just tried to take it as it came, and apart from the scare early on, we weren't overly worried throughout. As this baby had taken 18 months to create, the fear of losing it was so much greater, not only as of course no one wants to lose a baby, but also the thought of if we did would it take us another 18 months or longer to get pregnant again? I spoke to the doctor to confirm our pregnancy and ask what I should do about the Fertility Clinic referral she had kindly made, and she said as it was still early days (and because of the x-rays) when the referral came through I should make an appointment, and see how everything was a couple of days beforehand.

I followed her advice and managed to book a date for what would be just after the 12 weeks (and hopefully once a scan had confirmed everything was progressing as it should be). I also prepared for another bleed around the 6 week mark as we had experienced the last time, and sure enough, the pain and bleeding started on week 5+5 days. This time I tried not to worry as it had happened last time, and everything had been ok. I managed to get the doctor to refer me to the EPAS clinic and we had a scan 3 days later. Thankfully once again whilst they could see the bleed, our baby was still there and it's little heart beating strongly away. I asked what could cause these bleeds (as they were heavy, painful bleeds, not the implantation spotting we are warned may happen around this stage), and the midwife said I may have damage to my cervix; she also found a cyst on my left ovary which could have played a part in our fertility issues, which they said they would check on at the 12-week scan.

As I write this today I have just reached the 24-week milestone, our foetus is officially a baby (although it always has been to us since the moment we found out about it). I am grateful for every day, and do not take any of it for granted. This pregnancy has been slightly overshadowed by the current COVID-19 scare, and I am on week 4 of 12 weeks self-isolation. My husband is having to miss out on all of the appointments and scans as partners are no longer allowed to attend appointments (I completely understand why but it is still sad). We had also hoped to take our son along to one of the scans (I have monthly growth scans due to our first little one being so tiny when born even though he was overdue, and the fact that his growth stopped towards the end). My concerns now are to stay healthy for the remainder of this pregnancy, and that my husband will be allowed to attend the birth – if not I'll just keep my legs closed and refuse to push... as I remember it, it's totally within my control, right? Haha!

I fully appreciate whilst writing this that my experiences with periods, fertility and pregnancy have, compared to some people's journeys and heartbreak, been relatively straight forward; nonetheless, they have left their mark on me both physically and emotionally. I am so grateful for my son (as bloody hard as parenting can be sometimes – especially in lockdown!), and I am also so grateful for the love and support of my amazing husband who spent years rubbing my back and holding my hair back whilst I threw up during the bad periods; was so physically and emotionally supportive after the birth of our son when I couldn't be the wife I wanted to be; who supported me through the brief 18 months of sadness whilst we tried for a second baby.

My heart goes out to every female who has or is struggling with painful or heavy periods, who is missing school/work, feels embarrassed from leaks on clothes or furniture, and isn't being taken seriously when she goes to the doctors to explain her struggles; for every female who has tried multiple forms of contraceptive (either to help manage painful periods, or who just didn't want a baby at that precise moment in time), and has struggled with wild hormonal shifts, weight gain, breakthrough bleeding, or other nasty side effects (one of my school friends sadly had a blood clot as a result of the pill, nearly died, and has suffered from multiple health complications ever since); to every female who has tried to conceive and has felt the disappointment of a negative pregnancy test; for every female who has put themselves through the pains of various fertility treatments, to either be successful, or to once again experience the disappointment of a negative test, or a positive one followed by the unimaginable pain of a miscarriage. My heart goes out to them all, not only as it is all exhausting and a physical and emotional drain, but also that in many cases it is made so much worse by a lack of understanding (or caring) on behalf of some medical professionals. I think it is wonderful that women are opening up about the subjects of periods, fertility and miscarriages, which for too long have been seen as taboo subjects, or something which we should be ashamed of. We all have stories, whether minor like mine, or heart-breaking like several of my dear friends, but by talking and sharing our stories we can hopefully help and support our friends and family who may be silently going through similar situations.

Fran

Fran sought solace in family when she felt at her lowest with Hyperemesis Gravidarum, and felt guilt about feeling ill around her daughter.

Hello! I'm Fran and I'm 30. I live in Shrewsbury and am a stay at home mum to my (almost) 3 year old daughter Ivy. My husband Llewelyn works away Monday-Friday so I solo-parent a lot of the time!

When I was pregnant in 2017 with Ivy, I suffered from and was diagnosed with Hyperemesis Gravidarum (pregnancy sickness) and put on a course of tablets. I was sick up to 5/6 times a day and had lots of time off work (SEN TA at the time) but was able to rest, and by 12ish weeks it was mostly gone. Fast forward to 2019 and pregnant with daughter number 2. Around 9 weeks I began again with severe sickness. I was unable to keep anything down, even water, and was being sick up to 7 times daily (which for HG is still fairly minimal!). Throughout this time, I felt absolutely miserable. I was bed-bound a lot of the time because movement made me worse, and I was so weak from not eating. I couldn't even walk into my kitchen without throwing up. I was scared to leave the house as every bout of sickness was so severe, it would cause me to wet myself also. I was still being sick until I was around 20weeks, even though I was on medication that "worked". Even on the tablets, which I would take at bedtime every day, I still felt nauseous most days. I stopped taking them at 33 weeks when a doctor rang and said I shouldn't be taking them in my 3rd trimester, which was news to me!! The whole experience really affected my daughter, who's very switched on for her age. She was seeing mummy being sick and crying every day, and got very anxious by this. In turn, her sleep was affected, and her general mood. Even now when she's role playing with her dollies, they're always "sick" or "poorly" which makes me feel awful!! It's made the whole pregnancy experience really horrible to be honest, and I always feel so guilty for saying it as I know I'm extremely lucky.

I tried various different medications but none worked. I was finally prescribed a new medication which seemed to do the trick, when I was around 11weeks pregnant.

Ivy was amazing at getting into a routine of bringing me water and rubbing my back when I was sick, or shouting for daddy/Nannie when they were around. It became the norm for her, unfortunately.

Llewelyn was a fantastic help at weekends when he was here, and entertained Ivy so I could rest, in between making sure I was drinking plenty and eating what I could.

My mum and dad were absolute godsends and would take Ivy to the park/on walks etc when I wasn't able to, and just generally looked after me. Wetting myself whilst being sick/crying hysterically in front of my dad was a real low point, but he was un-phased!

I have some amazing friends who have been a fantastic support to me also!

My emotions whilst pregnant are very up and down anyway, and it was hard to snap out of feeling fairly depressed most days when I was at my worst. Not a lot helped on those days to be honest! Relationships were also a little strained - I felt like the worst mum to Ivy for months as I just couldn't do anything with her! She still tells me she loves me about a million times a day though and we're back to normal life now thankfully, until her sister arrives!!! My relationship with Llewelyn never really changes - he's a brilliant support to me, even when I'm miserable and snappy!

Unfortunately, I have associated a lot of things that I watched at the time, with feeling sick. I mean it was mostly The Wiggles, Room on the Broom, The Gruffalo....you get the gist! I was housebound with a toddler! However sick these make me feel now, these programmes were a godsend at the time to keep Ivy entertained.

Music in general is my life, and I'll always whack on a bit of Spice Girls when I'm feeling low!

Helen

Helen had known for a long time that she would use a donor to help her conceive and has had support from professionals, friends and family alike.

I'm Helen, 39, mama to 2.5year old Olive and from Guernsey. I am one of 4 siblings and have 7 nieces and nephews. Kids have always been high on my agenda, but unfortunately, relationships haven't featured quite so highly, or worked, for whatever reason.

To become a mum by using a donor has been something I considered doing, right back to my early 20s - I have never wanted to contemplate that I would not have kids. I was relieved to have a positive conversation about this with my own mum when I was in my late 20s, so I decided then that I would try around 34 years if I hadn't met anyone. She admitted that she would have done the same had she not met my dad, so was fully behind me - even though she tried to nudge the age to 36. Mum passed away a couple of years later.

I was fortunate enough to have a couple of contacts with some knowledge on the subject, a cousin who had done the same, and a same-sex couple who had used the same process. This was incredibly helpful as much of the investigation into options had been done for me, so it didn't take me long to decide to use Cryos, a Danish sperm bank. With the help of a couple of close friends, I made a shortlist of potential donors - there is quite a lot of detail available and you can narrow it down to suit your preferences.

Initially I tried hopefully with home insemination, several times, but to no avail. So I started to prepare myself for IVF. Honestly, this was tricky and a real juggle around work - I had to know that I could leave the island at short notice, all the while trying not to tell anyone. I was, perhaps, ill-prepared the first time and it was an interesting ride. Several scans during the process were required over here, and this in itself can be difficult to arrange and quite stressful. A baseline scan on day 2 or 3 of my cycle and, once confirmed with the clinic that everything was as needed, injections started, then another a few days later, and one more - at which point the clinic confirm the appointment dates in Denmark. Unfortunately, I had been on a high dose for the hormone stimulation, and experienced overstimulated ovaries. So, while they harvested a high number of eggs, it was painful and I felt rotten. I was swollen and bloated, dehydrated, and felt quite sick. I was also in Denmark alone - so it was all a bit strange. They successfully placed one embryo back in my uterus before I returned home, but I was quite unwell for several days and the swelling took a long time to subside. I had a positive test result at 14 days post transfer but unfortunately miscarried a couple of weeks later.

Five months later, I returned to Denmark, having juggled work commitments and appointments once again. I felt better prepared, I knew what was coming and I was well hydrated, less stimulated and had a friend join me for a few days. Everything went much more smoothly and this was the cycle that resulted in my daughter arriving in August 2017. I had expected mixed reactions to my pregnancy and circumstances, but thankfully if anyone had any negative thoughts, they didn't vocalise them in my direction and I received nothing but support. Around 3 months after Olive arrived, I realised that I was suffering from some form of PND, I recognised it by my loss of appetite - I am very slim and can't afford to lose weight. I wasn't feeling sad, just a bit grey, and having a lot of anxious thoughts. My doctor was very supportive and I started taking anti-depressants which thankfully lifted me out of it. It surprised me as I found the first 3 months fairly easy, but it just crept up.

Being one of four, I always wanted four myself, but I am realistic and I know that this isn't going to be the case for me now. However, I really would like Olive to have a sibling, someone in the same boat as her, and hopefully a good friend to go through life with, whether I am around for many years or not.

In 2019 I tried one home insemination, but as of June 2019 this was not an option as the Danish laws changed so that donor sperm can't be sent to private residential addresses, and nowhere here on Guernsey will perform IUI with donor sperm - so IVF (or IUI off-island) was my only option. I went through it all again and went to Denmark in November, with my sister and my cousin each joining for a few days to help out with the toddler in tow. All went fine and one embryo was transferred - but unfortunately an early scan revealed issues and on 22nd December I had to have a laparoscopy as this was an ectopic pregnancy. I hadn't really thought this might happen as they place the embryo in the uterus, but I know now that they can drift, which is what happened. So, under general anaesthetic (which terrified me), one fallopian tube was removed and I was sent home to recover. Emotionally, I was feeling pretty rotten, but I am quite pragmatic and recognise how lucky I was that the scan showed this and that I didn't end up with a ruptured tube and a far worse fate. I was fortunate that there were 3 embryos frozen on this round of IVF so I remain hopeful and cross my fingers that when the COVID19 situation has passed, I can try to use one of these and have a sibling for Olive. Time will tell.

I feel incredibly lucky to have a wonderful support network. Solo parenting isn't for the faint hearted - I am her everything, 24/7 and it's honestly exhausting some days. Not having someone to bounce off and share the little moments with is hard, but she doesn't know any different and we have a lot of family around us. I haven't tried to pursue any relationships since she arrived, and I don't intend to for the time being, but I would love to meet someone in the future. It's not easy to meet anyone as a solo parent though as, unlike separated parents, we don't have nights and days off without roping in babysitters/friends/family - so I will climb that mountain when it comes to it! There are quite a lot of people on social media who I follow now who have done the same, it's nice to have a little virtual network of people who "get it".

www.facebook.com/helen.young.581

Jane

Jane will never forget the two babies she lost at various stages of pregnancy but her family is now completed with Kate and Hatty, her grown-up daughters, and her husband Sion.

I'm Jane. I grew up in Herefordshire but left at 18 to go to university. I spent 3 years in Newcastle and 2 years living in Germany before moving to Cardiff to become a teacher. I stayed in Cardiff for 40 years and then moved to Guernsey a year ago to join my husband who had already been working there for a year. Despite having been lucky enough to have had a fulfilled and mostly happy life, at the age of 65 I am still haunted by feelings of loss and "what ifs" and "if onlys".

I met my first long-term partner, Tudor, when I was 19 and we led a fairly selfish life doing pretty much what we wanted with children not high on my agenda. I didn't feel particularly maternal or broody. I got to the age of 32 and my partner suggested we should maybe think about having a baby. I still didn't feel particularly maternal but thought we should give it a go. It was not long before I found out I was pregnant- and I was terrified. Could I be a good mum? Could I love a baby? My relationship was not going well and I was beset by feelings of doubt and downright fear, Then, on 21st December 1987 my beautiful daughter Kate, a little bundle of total perfection was born after a long and very difficult labour with the cord round her neck. After a brief hello she was rushed off to the special baby unit and my life was changed forever. I had never felt such love. I felt overwhelmed and consumed by it and have never felt such relief as when she came out of SBU.

My relationship sadly broke down and I became a single parent, which was no hardship. I treasured every moment I could spend with her. Then when she was 4 I met Sion, my husband. I was 37 by then and we soon knew we were really keen to have a baby together. I thought it would be easy and when I got pregnant at 40 it didn't occur to me that things could get tough. The pregnancy was quite hard. I felt sick and exhausted all the time, but was kept going by the thought of the beautiful baby at the end of it. I tried to carry on as normal, still doing my dance classes and going to gigs as long as I could sit down! I will never forget the Bon Jovi gig in Cardiff Arms Park. We got moved into the VIP enclosure and Holly kicked and danced along all the way through. "I will always love you" became her song. Then when I was 34 weeks pregnant I could not feel a heartbeat and lost a bit of blood. My wonderful GP came and sent me to hospital "just to be on the safe side." I will never forget the concerned midwife, Lorna, who had to send for someone more senior and then those words, "I am sorry to have to tell you that sometime between Saturday and today your baby has died." The words would not sink in, but then I realised that I would have to go through labour to give birth to my dead baby. I felt guilty- guilty that I had not been able to protect her and afraid- afraid of what she would look like. I am so glad I gave birth to our perfect little Holly with Sion at my side and being my rock all the way through. She was born on 3rd October 1995 at 9.12, weighing 3lbs 14 oz. She was the most perfect, gorgeous baby and we kept hoping against hope that she would open her eyes. She never did though and we had to somehow struggle on without her. I don't know how we managed the funeral, but we buried a sunflower with her, which became our symbol of hope. Sion carried her tiny white casket and I somehow managed to read the poem "Spring morning" by A A Milne. It was such a tough day, but we had both managed to do one last thing for our precious baby.

No-one knew what to say to us and we clung together, trying to comfort each other, but each drowning in our own grief and disappointment. I had a lot more support than Sion and I didn't realise until much later how hard it had been for him to come to terms with the loss of our beautiful baby. Fathers often get forgotten.

I was lucky enough to get pregnant again in 1996, but was unable to feel the joy and excitement that I had felt with Holly. I was constantly on edge and even when the 12 week scan showed everything to be normal, I had little faith that things would turn out well. Then, at 16 weeks I was due to have an amniocentesis test, but when we had our consultation, the doctor said the baby wasn't growing as normal. My fears had been founded and I was sent home with a tablet to bring on miscarriage and told to go back the next day- I didn't last that long though. I started miscarrying at home and Sion had to rush me back to hospital. It was a very frightening experience but I could feel nothing. I didn't even find out the sex of our second lost baby, but we were both convinced that it as a boy, who we would have called Patrick. I felt numb and hopeless. The empty arms are so painful.

We kept trying for me to get pregnant again, but I think psychologically I had shut down and couldn't cope with yet more loss. Then, a year later we decided to have a go at IVF. We knew that the chances of success were slim given my age, but it was worth one more go. We spent our savings and went to Bristol for treatment. We managed to get 3 eggs and I forced myself to be positive, but as predicted, my period arrived and we had to accept that this was probably not going to end happily, however many attempts we had.

I tried to put the feelings of loss and failure to the back of my mind and we went on lots of holidays and tried to enjoy life with my beautiful Kate, but the empty arms kept hurting and we started to talk about adoption.

In 2001 we decided to start the process to adopt. It was long, gruelling and intrusive, but in 2002 we were approved to adopt a child and in July 2002 18 month old Hatty joined our family. She was fierce, feisty and independent and so in need of love. The empty arms were filled, but she hasn't replaced Holly or our second lost baby. She was and is a person in her own right. She brought us so much joy and her mischief as a little girl definitely kept us on our toes. It has been a difficult journey and her adolescent years have been very troubled but she is so loved.

As I look back and reflect, Kate is 32 and Hatty is 20- she is still not out of the woods, but I feel so lucky to have had 2 beautiful girls to love and care for. I have never forgotten my other 2 babies and often wonder and ask all the "What ifs", but life throws us curve balls and we have to do what we can to survive them. "I will always love you" no longer makes me cry, but brings a smile to my lips. The baskets of flowers I have learned to arrange for birthdays and anniversaries, which always contain sunflowers are life-affirming, as is sitting in the peace of the cemetery. The books I read, such as "Love, Labour and Loss" and "Continuing Bonds" and my consequent interest in psychology and counselling led to further study and new qualifications which meant I have been able to help others.

I have been lucky in so many ways. I will never forget and some days, often unexpectedly, can still be difficult, but I am so glad to have loved and the loss has taught me a lot about the power of love and the strength of the human spirit.

Kayleigh

Kayleigh was tested throughout her pregnancy for diabetes, was asked questions about safeguarding and her daughter stopped moving as much toward the end of her pregnancy.

Before I start writing my pregnancy experience, I would like to introduce myself and give you an idea of who I am. I will be writing as if I am talking to you in person in a busy coffee shop treating myself to a latte and a cookie. So here goes...

I am a 30-year-old Salopian, born in Shrewsbury (UK) surrounded by the beautiful Shropshire Hills that inspired J. R. R Tolkien, where Charles Darwin grew up and known as the 'town of flowers'. Shropshire is a beautiful part of the world and I currently live here with my husband, beautiful daughter and my little zoo of gerbils and rabbits. Work-wise, I specialize in education where I have taught and supported students in a variety of settings including SEN, SEMH, residential, and mainstream schools. Now I am thinking of a career change but that's a conversation for another time, so let's get onto pregnancy!

My hubby and I wanted children so decided at the end of January 2019 to plan, so I came off the combined pill and within a month I became pregnant. I didn't really feel anything till March as I started to feel sickly and I was due my period, so I got a pregnancy test and the result was positive. At this time, we were living in a one 1st floor flat and had little room for ourselves let a room for a baby so looking for bigger accommodation was on the 'to do' list.

I showed my husband the result and his reply was 'yay...oh shit', because he knew we had a lot to sort out and to tell our parents. You are probably thinking why is that an issue? It wasn't an issue but the previous year we got married and the previous year we started dating. Everything clicked and felt right, so we went with it and here we are now preparing for a baby.

My family and friends were over the moon, but my hubby's parents' reaction was shock and we aren't sure why, but it was.

March 2019. We are a few weeks in, so we decided to go and get a private scan because the first NHS scan was week 11 or 12 of pregnancy and I didn't want to wait that long because of the type of work I was doing at the time. We thought we were 4 weeks in but we were actually 7 weeks in and I started to show after 2 months! My in-laws thought I had put on weight because they said I shouldn't be showing so early, but you know what? Your body is different to everyone else's and you can show at any point, so the one shoe size fits all phrase is a load of bollocks.

April – June 2019. The busiest time of our lives here, because we had to get cars that were deemed as safe and we moved to a new house. This was pure chaos and we managed with the support of our friends and family. At this time, I had none of the typical pregnancy symptoms such as throwing up, cravings, backache etc.... The one thing I did have throughout was acid reflux and it occurred during the whole day.

*Tip: drink soda water. It's cheap and you can carry it around wherever you go without looking like you're a Gaviscon junkie. Acid flavoured tablets also work but only for so long.

Wonderful summertime. Yes, that lovely time of year in England where in 2019 it was actually bloody hot and I had to ninja myself around in the shade at work so I didn't cook my baby or become dehydrated. At this point, my feet were starting to swell and I couldn't drink enough water to help it, so regular breaks were needed, and I felt useless at work. I am an independent person who likes to be on the go, keeping busy and helping others but it was becoming harder as the weeks went by. It was becoming frustrating for me and I had to accept growing a little human takes a lot of energy and I had to listen to my body, otherwise karma would pay me a visit!

At the end of the summer, my job was coming to an end. It was contracted term time and I knew it would be difficult to find another job. I never reapplied for the role because I realized towards the end it wasn't for me and it's okay to say that regardless of the circumstances, so I finished my job and went on job seekers allowance as I still wanted to work whilst I could.

I am not ashamed I went on JSA but I applied to any job I thought I could do and knew that it would be incredibly difficult as I was heavily pregnant, but I was still capable of working.

In September and October, I worked as a temporary learning support assistant at a college, so I proved to myself and my family that you can get work if you really push for it and happy to do temporary work. At this time, I applied for maternity allowance and this was incredibly stressful because it took up to 10 weeks to find out whether I would get support or not. We found out at the end of November that I was accepted and the money per month was just under £600, which covered my bills and shopping which relieved my husband of supporting me a bit.

Throughout my pregnancy, I was tested for Gestational diabetes because my BMI was high and in every test I came out clear, but towards the end, my hormones went haywire and sugar levels went all over the shop so they asked me to test my blood on a daily basis. We found out that bread in the morning was the trigger, but I could eat 3 crumpets with jam and my sugar levels were fine. Bizarre isn't it?

This caused me the most stress because the consultant basically said I was more likely to get type 2 diabetes and this that and the other. I didn't need this on top of them asking about any safeguarding issues in front of my husband during the third trimester. The safeguarding question is about any concerns you have about neighbours, family members or friends. Now, my problem with this is that they asked me twice in front of my husband with a student doctor present. This made my husband feel incredibly uncomfortable and started to question how he appeared to others, his behaviour and communication. If you ever met my husband, he is not the most social person in the world, but he has a heart of gold and came to every appointment with me. I couldn't have asked for a better husband who was helping to build a family home and prepare for our baby to arrive.

When we had the home visits we mentioned our consultations to the midwives, as it happened on more than one occasion and they were not happy with how it left us feeling, so they took it back to their managers and hopefully something has been done about it.

In the last two months of pregnancy, our daughter decided to be lazy and not move as much, so I went to triage about 3 or 4 times and it's always best to get checked out. When I had to test my sugar levels, I had to pop into the hospital to pick up more slides and needles, so they moved my growth scan on the same day and I mentioned I hadn't felt much movement. Well! During the growth scan, there was barely any amniotic fluid around our baby and the lady was deeply concerned, so they shipped me off to Triage to double-check on our baby's movement and my consultant came in to see me. I cannot forget her words 'If your baby does not move enough we will induce you tonight, but if she moves I would like to induce you tomorrow as I am concerned about the lack of fluid around your baby.'

Like, holy hot cakes! Seriously!? I wasn't due for another two weeks but we knew the little lady would come early. We just had that feeling and you should always go with your gut feeling no matter what anyone else tells you. So, bubba is moving fine and we were relieved that I wasn't being induced that evening but we knew we had a mad panic when we got home to sort the last little bits out because I was due in the next day at 10 AM (eek!).

The following day, we were both feeling okay, putting myself in the mindset that I am going to run a physical and emotional marathon because that's exactly how you must see it. You need to have that mental state of knowing it's going to be long and your body will do what it needs to do to get this baby out. The midwives are there to monitor and guide you whilst keeping you and the baby safe.

So, we are now in the pre-labour ward and I have quite a few Midwives asking about my diet and to be honest about it, so I tell them... I eat fairly well, I don't snack, I don't smoke, or drink and I exercise but probably enough to shift a few pounds. At this point I was walking my parents' dog twice a day for 30 minutes each time, still driving and being active where possible. The more midwives asked me the more I got annoyed and told them I am fully aware of why they are asking me, but it won't change the current circumstances so back off. What annoyed them even more was that my blood pressure was perfect and went against their textbook. Oh yes, thanks to doing martial arts for 12 years my blood pressure was and still is better than most peoples.

A lady came to me talking about a trial where they are researching to find ways to help induce early labour without any chemical and if we opted to participate it was a 50% chance we would be chosen for this non-chemical inducement or have the usual drip and force labour to occur.

We were chosen for the non-chemical trial and five flat biro like sticks were inserted. It was uncomfortable but bearable. I was walking like John Wayne for a few hours and when it came to the loo, well, you had to imagine you were going to sit on an invisible horse and slowly lower yourself down. Whilst I was doing this I could imagine reverse lights and beeping going on in my head because it took a while getting used to and the fact I nominated myself up for this trial, which only prolonged my labour and kept me in hospital longer!

After 16 hours the Doctor and supporting Midwife took out what now looked like small glue gun sticks. Luckily it wasn't uncomfortable when they took them out. They didn't wait the full 24 hours because I couldn't feel any contractions, but my cervix did dilate without any pain. Go me. The midwives decided to move me up to the labour ward, hook me up to a drip and break my waters. I have got to say having your waters broke is not pleasant and I found it the most painful part of my labour. No joke.

My advice here would be to take the gas and air, because it does take away the pain and you need to take long, deep breaths but not too many to make you space out.

So, my waters are broken, and they ramp up my drip to full because I couldn't feel my contractions despite, I was having them and could see them on the monitor. Within 4 hours I went from 0 to 5CM. During this time, I was walking round in a baggy t-shirt and my underwear without a care in the world. The only people in the room were my husband and my midwife Kate, who was lovely and chatty.

When my contractions finally started getting stronger, I could feel a tingle in my lower back and eventually this became more intense to the point you can't talk when it occurs. When the pain really started to kick in, I would close my eyes and focus on my breathing.

This is important during your whole labour because you don't know how long it is going to be and you need to stay in control, but flow with your contractions as you need to relax. Easier said than done but don't fight against your body, your body knows what it is doing, and you just need to help it to get your baby out.

After ramping up my medication to start my labour I start vomiting as I contracted, and this was hard between a sip of water and taking gas and air. Personally, I did not want an epidural because I've got a history of a bad back and didn't want any further problems in the future.

Another useful tip here, get your partner, doula or support network to hold a cup of water in one hand and the gas in the other. Discuss before your labour that you will nod to which one you want. This worked well for me during labour and my husband was on it.

Also, during my first few hours of labour, I get the shakes and feel incredibly cold then I become very hot. My husband and Midwife Kate were probably toasting their socks off, but my body was going into shock and reacting to labour. So, between vomiting, gas and drinking water, I was peeing as I was contracting and once I got to 6CM's because I wanted to push but I was told not to.

This became harder as my cervix dilated further and I had my eyes closed for most of the time. I had my back turned to the midwife and was holding my husbands' hand. He was checking in on me asking if I was okay but didn't make any unnecessary chit chat because it wasn't needed. He supported me by reminding me not to push, to keep breathing and continue drinking water.

At some point, I was given anti-vomiting medication to help me cope because I couldn't keep the water down and I needed fluid throughout. Once I reached 6CM's they reduced the drug that induces your labour as I was well into my labour now. At this point, my Midwife completed her shift and swapped with Midwife Stephanie.

I can't say I thought of much during my labour. I just listened to my body, breathed and took water or gas when I needed it. The only thing I said to myself in my head was 'it is like a marathon; you just need to pace yourself and stay calm. You are in control and you are in safe hands. Keep going.'

It is so important to mentally prepare yourself. This does not mean to go and read every single article out there, although I have to say I did, because I'm a little bit nerdy when it comes to learning new things and what current studies are showing.

At 10CM's Stephanie said I was ready to push our baby out (remember we still don't know the gender) and she told me when she says push to push three times then have a break. A little bit like reps, one rep of three pushes and they had to be good strong pushes, so my advice is to take a deep breath and push whilst you breathe out.

The ring of fire did not bother me, and it only stung a little, because at this point you want the baby out. I had peed myself so many times and the poor ladies had to put essentially puppy pads under my ass. I was tired of vomiting, the gas and air had made me a little giddy, but mostly I was sweaty and desperately needed a shower.

Eventually, our baby arrived, a beautiful girl and our lives changed forever.

One chapter ends and another one starts.

www.facebook.com/kayleigh.bowden1

Lell

I'm Eleanor, but to family and friends, and for the purposes of the book, I'm Lell. Diagnosed with secondary infertility, I try to explain the vicious circles I endure and the endless questions I ask myself.

I'm 35 years old, from Herefordshire, am married, have a 4 year old son and a cat called Rufio.

It took 2 years and 3 months of 'trying' to get pregnant with Wilf. I use inverted commas with that word because some months we definitely tried harder. Some months we'd try just once and then cross our fingers, other times we'd have sex 5 times around ovulating, I'd lie with my legs stuck up in the air, eat lots of healthy food, take vitamins, avoid caffeine, do a fertility dance... you know of the things I refer to. For the most part, it was a world where I followed a repetitive and emotional cycle; wee on a stick, wee on a stick, ovulate, have sex, wait for 2 long weeks, start period, be grumpy. Repeat.

On the months we didn't do much, I blamed us for not trying harder. On the months where we were trying hard, in so many ways, I berated myself for stressing about it too much. I wondered what was wrong. Whether *I* was wrong. One of the reasons we left Herefordshire was to work in a less stressful place to see if that helped. It did not. I went to my GP after a year of trying, and her response was, 'It's a bit early to see me.' Gee, thanks. 12

months of the vicious cycle wasn't enough for her. I continued for another 6 months then went back, to be given a blood test and for Adam to be asked for a sperm sample. Everything came back fine, which was infuriating.

I gave up booze (not for 2 years I hasten to add, but I did give it up for a while!), I tried meditation, I stopped eating meat because I heard that helped. Still nothing.

Then one night, after a lot of wine, it happened. I got pregnant. I remember being back in Herefordshire that Easter and just not wanting to drink wine or tea and thinking that was really unusual. When I was late for my period, I couldn't believe it, in fact I left it another week and a half before I told Adam and did a test because I just couldn't believe it to be true.

I am hugely grateful that I had a fairly straightforward pregnancy. The birth I'll talk about another time, but all three of us are happy and healthy, give or take a minor addiction to chocolate.

For various reasons: the birth, the colic and the anxiety after Wilf was born, I swore never to have another child. I imagine many other mothers have said the same, in fact I know they have. I swore we'd adopt in those early days. So I started looking into it. But this was only brief; we just sort of got on with life as it was. It wasn't until Wilf turned 2 that I thought 'OK, I can do this. Let's have another baby'. Rose-tinted glasses and all that.

So, I came off the pill and the process started again. The month I write this marks 2 years and 3 months of trying, but this time we're still not pregnant. I've been to the GP (a nicer one this time round!) because not only am I not pregnant but my periods are awful. She was sympathetic and wonderful. Sent me for blood tests straight away, referred me to an osteopath "it'll help you relax" she said! She also sent me to a consultant. She'd indicated he'd want to do scans when I saw him, which I was nervous about and made sure all areas of hairiness were immaculate (a good friend who'd also been to see him said not to bother - he's seen all manner of vulva and he wouldn't bat an eyelid). Anyway, he did no scans at all which was beyond disappointing as I was hoping for an immediate "You can't have any more kids, your uterus is closed for business" or, perhaps more annoyingly, "all is well - keep going!" Instead, he has referred me to the hospital 3 months from then to have an HSG which is a series of x-rays taken while dye is squirted into the uterus to see where it goes and whether the fallopian tubes are blocked. I was of course, terrified. Mostly because he said "Take some antibiotics in case you catch chlamydia" and "Bring pain killers - some women really feel it." Thanks mate. (As you can tell, I have white-coat phobia and am scared of everything!)

However, now COVID-19 is rife and we're in lockdown, any chance of that happening is over for a good while anyway.

What was frustrating was that it was all on me. It must be *my tubes* that are blocked or *my uterus* that is grumpy. Rather than anything being down to Adam.

The consultant also prescribed me some drugs that had DO NOT TAKE IF YOU'RE TRYING TO GET PREGNANT plastered on the side. I mean, honestly.

But it leaves me back at square 1, although I've ditched the ovulation tests now because I think it was winding me up more than I needed them to. But now I play the guessing game 'Is my discharge like an egg white today? Do I feel slightly warmer today?' Ridiculous triggers to look for.

I've tried really hard again - no booze, folic acid, extra spinach and avocado, not having my laptop anywhere near my crotch. I've tried not caring again - which of course is my favourite. (Please refrain from saying 'just relax' to a person trying to get pregnant, it actually doesn't help). And every month so far, I end up disappointed, angry, sad, confused.

So where has it left me? Feeling guilty and incredibly tearful that I've wasted so much time thinking about having another kid when I have a perfectly hilarious and gorgeous creature already. I feel that I've almost missed a year of Wilf because I've been so focused and almost obsessed with something else. On the flip side, I've felt excited that this could be a family of 3 and we can afford holidays, hobbies and focus on a healthy work/life/parent balance. But gutted that Wilf won't spend Christmas surrounded by siblings. Guilt again that I'm using holidays as a plus point.

I'm really nervous about the idea of surgery and can't afford the time or money or perhaps even further heartache for IVF. Adoption we talk about, but we don't think it's for us. How long do we keep trying for? Is it worth suffering such long periods between ovulation?! Can we just embrace the triangle family? These are the questions to consider this Summer.

The things that have helped most have been people. My husband is wonderful. He rolls with what happens and I'm hugely grateful for him. My friends and family; why didn't I open up about all this to them earlier!? The last 6 months I have talked more openly about everything and it is such a relief to do so - thank you to all of them! Going to the nice GP really helped and I know I could go back if I needed. Finding a supportive GP is super important.

Reading has been great. *It's About Bloody Time* by Emma Barnett is an absolute must-read for anyone who has had, is having, or is in the general vicinity of anyone who has periods. *One and Only* confirmed for me that it is totally OK to have just 1 child.

Also pages 187-189 of Becoming by Michelle Obama. It resonated beautifully at the time I read it and my gosh that woman is fab.

And of course Wilf. He brings joy to my heart and an ache in my face and if it's only him I ever have then I am the luckiest person.

I'm starting to appreciate that choosing not to have IVF is an acceptable choice, that a family of 3 will be lovely, and that the stigma of the 'only child' needs to be broken. I just need to own how I feel and not compare myself to anyone else.

"...*whatever good or bad fortune may come our way we can always give it meaning and transform it into something of value.*"
Hermanne Hesse, *Siddharta.*

Leonie

Leonie would like a sibling for her son, but has secondary infertility, so has turned to IVF before and during the pandemic.

My husband and I married in 2014. Like many couples, we were keen to start building our family soon after and we were lucky enough to conceive within six months.

We always wanted a sibling (or two) for our son and when he was 1.5 years old, we decided this would be a good time in our lives to further expand our family. My husband and I both have a 2 year gap with our siblings and we wanted to recreate this with our family.

At this point, I was aged 32 and my husband, 36. We were both fit and healthy and had no reasons to believe that another conception would be an issue.

A year on and nothing had happened. I decided to leave my nursing job as I felt the stress was a contribution to our fertility issues and we started the process of tests through the GP. About the same time, I started experiencing cyclical pain on my right side. The GP referred me for a scan but it was normal so a referral to gynaecology was made. By the time I had the appointment months later, I had daily pelvic pain and endometriosis was suspected. It took 9 months to get a laparoscopy and that was with me making two complaints about the waiting list times. Mild endometriosis was found but the doctors felt it was not affecting my fertility. They suspect it could be controlled by hormones but because I am trying to conceive, this is not an option at present so unfortunately, I have to live with the pain.

Whilst waiting for the laparoscopy, two years had passed since we had started trying and so we had decided to start the process of IVF (ICSI). I was 34 by this point and the doctors were confident with our chances. I remember feeling nervous anticipation; despite all the medication and their side-effects, the scans and egg collection and subsequent transfer, I believed it would bring us closer to having a baby. Unfortunately round one was unsuccessful and I was heartbroken and felt lost. We were lucky enough to have two frozen embryos and were able to make plans for them once I had recovered from my laparoscopy.

Sadly, both of my subsequent frozen embryo transfers resulted in early miscarriage and a chemical pregnancy. I bled both times from my "Official Test Day" and although the first pregnancy managed to hold on for a few weeks, the second one only lasted a matter of days. The doctor felt we had just been unlucky but suggested some further testing for recurrent miscarriage

Finally, after a few more months of waiting for the recurrent miscarriage test results, they came back normal so we got all geared up for another fresh cycle of IVF. Unfortunately, my cycle got cancelled due to the closure of clinics because of the Coronavirus pandemic. I struggled with all the waiting and not knowing when the fertility clinics would re-open and desperately wrote to the HFEA, my MP and my clinic for more clarification.

A few months later, we were pleased when the clinics started to re-open again. This involved another long protocol fresh cycle. Another couple of months of scans, injections, egg collection and waiting.

Unfortunately because of the pandemic, my husband was not able to attend the clinic so it made the process feel even more one-sided. I am lucky he was able to support me in other ways. This time we had one embryo transferred and another one frozen. Another two week wait and another positive pregnancy test but unfortunately this one was not to be either, only lasting a few days. It should have been the month my baby was due from my second embryo transfer and another 9 months on and I've still made no progress.

I am consumed by the world of infertility/ IVF and now, pregnancy loss. My life consists of scheduling and attending appointments, ultrasound scans, blood tests, injections, sorting prescriptions, side-effects from all the hormones. I can mostly cope with the physical discomfort from IVF but I struggle with all the emotional aspects. One of the most challenging parts is after egg collection, finding out if any eggs have fertilised, and then having to wait for phone calls to see if any of them make it to day 5 for embryo transfer. It is torture. And then comes the even longer "two week wait" before test day arrives, wondering if the symptoms are from the hormones, PMT or pregnancy. There is a lot about infertility that can't be controlled but I try and control what I am able to, such as my lifestyle choices, food and drink, exercise, self-care and mind-set.

Secondary infertility is a lonely place to be. I don't feel I fully belong in the "infertility club" as I am already a mother and cannot possibly comprehend the devastation of being unable to conceive a child, like many couples. I feel guilt that I should be happy with one child, as I am often reminded. However, I love my child with every fibre of my being so why wouldn't I want to create another one? I feel grief that infertility has detracted from my enjoyment as a mother to my son. I am enormously grateful to be a mum but it does not stop my maternal desire for a bigger family. It gives me enormous sadness that he is an only child and watching him play all alone for months over lockdown was a massive reminder of this. I am aware that if we have another child, the age-gap will be 5+ years now, so he will still be unlikely to have a play-mate. We are lucky that he hasn't asked questions yet as to why all his friends have brothers and sisters but I am sure it won't be long. All around our struggles, our friends were getting pregnant, having babies and completing their families and I struggle to watch siblings play and interact without feeling heartache. Even nursery drop-offs, toddler groups and trips to the park have become an issue for me. Pregnancy and new life is everywhere and it is challenging; a constant reminder of what I am working towards and failing. I avoid group situations that are a trigger as much as possible. I have also unfollowed people on social media for similar reasons. I appreciate this can be controversial, but for me, my mental wellbeing has to be my priority. Lockdown has also provided me with some much needed solitude and time to live in the moment.

I've largely kept our journey on a "need to know" basis with family and close friends, because unless you've experienced it, it can be difficult to comprehend. I also don't want the additional pressure of others being in the "two week wait" with me. I've lost count of the number of people who have asked me when baby number two is coming and the myriad of emotion that brings for me behind closed doors; mostly a silent, enduring grief.

During my years dealing with infertility, I have used Facebook groups, which have been my lifeline for support and information. I moderate two infertility groups, which means I can use my experiences to help other women. I have also recently found my infertility family on Instagram; strong, inspiring women. I have found it so helpful to connect with women who understand. However, even within the "trying to conceive" community, it can feel like other women are making progress when my body is failing. Obviously, everyone's path is so individual and I need to remind myself of this and take a break from accounts when necessary. My husband doesn't use social media so only focuses on our journey, without the comparisons, but he doesn't get the emotional support I find so useful. I have made so many wonderful friends on this journey, for which, I will always be grateful. I have also utilised the counselling support offered at my fertility clinic, which offers a safe impartial space.

To cope with the journey, I make sure I take time out to do activities that I enjoy; that make me feel like me.

My husband and I try to ensure we have date nights and time for us. Meditation/mindfulness has become a big part of my life and I practice gratitude; there is so much to be thankful for.

We are now in the process of making a plan to use our final embryo. It is difficult to know whether we have just been unlucky so far, or if there are more tests we need to be considering.

Over time, it has been more difficult to imagine a happy ending. I am aware that there will come a point where IVF may become less statistically viable for us. The assumption is that infertility affects fertility. The reality is that it also affects marriage, friendships, finances, career, mental and physical health, sleep, weight, dietary intake; basically every aspect of life. These issues, as well as age, may eventually outweigh our ability to continue with fertility treatment. This scares me but for now, I just have to live in hope that whatever our outcome, we will find a way to accept and live our life to the full.

Since the time of starting to write this post, my final embryo transfer sadly ended in a 'missed' miscarriage. I am now undergoing more tests before completing our final fresh IVF cycle.

I remain hopeful yet realistic of our chance to bring home our baby.

If you want to follow my story, my Instagram is _ttc_a_sibling_for_t

Lil

Lil waited for what felt like 'a thousand years' before she met her beautiful daughter Olin. She knows it was worth the wait.

I'm Lisa, or Lil, I'm 45 next month and the unbelievably lucky mom to a 4-year-old pocket rocket!

My journey to meet Olin, my daughter, began when I was 36. Olin's dad and I had been together for 6 years and decided to try for a baby! I knew I was at that "tricky age" and it might take time but I'd no idea of the journey we were about to take...that would end four years later.

6 months after we began trying I was undergoing all kinds of tests to see why we hadn't fallen pregnant yet. We tried IUI numerous times and then decided IVF and ICSI was the route to take.

I was extremely fortunate to have sold a house and bought a house with my daughter's father...I kept some money aside for an IVF fund. Not everyone is this fortunate and due to my age, I knew I'd need to go all-in if I was going to go down this road...I wanted the funds available to enable us to try 3 rounds. That's what we could afford.

Journey one begins. A fresh round, of course...over stimulation, swollen tummy and the wind! No one tells you about the wind! I swear every step I took I could feel my ovaries bounce!!

We were fortunate enough to have lots of eggs retrieved, quite a few mature enough, 7 that fertilised and 5 that were good enough to use. 2 became day 5 blastocysts and 3 were day 3 embryos. One blasto was a "gold medalist" so we decided to have just one egg transferred.

Now, I have pretty good will power, so I waited exactly 14 days before I did the test and I didn't look at it but gave it to my boyfriend so he would be the first to know if we've had a positive result or not. It was positive! First try! How unbelievably lucky.

Unfortunately, within days I was bleeding and over an August weekend, I miscarried. It was utterly devastating no matter how much you think you are prepared that this could happen.

We tried again right away as we had frozen eggs so very soon after I was having 2 embryos transferred...! Again, I waited the 14 days and did the test and gave it to my boyfriend before I looked.

His face said it all, he didn't need to say anything. It was a failed attempt. I wasn't prepared for this at all and it really had an impact. It was just before Christmas so we decided to wait a few months before trying our last round. We still had a blasto and an embryo frozen and waiting!

We started our final round and I was much less hopeful and I felt so guilty about that...maybe it was self-deprivation. I'd be less disappointed when it didn't work, right?

So...I get a call from the clinic, although both eggs thawed perfectly...the embryo didn't survive...but the blasto was going strong! I'd only have one transferred.

I had the procedure on April 01st 2015...

Again...I waited the 14 days and did the test without looking at the results...I handed the test to my boyfriend and couldn't look at him and asked him to wait a moment before telling me the result as I didn't believe it had worked so wanted just a final moment before knowing I wasn't pregnant.

I should have had more faith. He waited a moment then told me it was positive!

I had a couple of scary moments during my pregnancy but it all turned out fine and I loved every moment. I met Olin, the love of my life, in the December.

Unfortunately, it was a really tough ride for us and our journey took its toll. When Olin was 18 months old, her father and I split up.

Olin was absolutely worth the wait.

I tear up when I hear Christina Perri "A Thousand Years"...those words. It's our song. I look at her often and can't quite believe she is here and I get to be her mommy.

www.facebook.com/lills.dodd

Lorna

Lorna offers some comprehensive views of miscarriage, including a more 'unexpected' reaction; one not of grief and sorrow, but of moving on and a form of gratitude. Which of course, is also ok.

My name is Lorna, I'm 36 and I live in The North with my husband and our very lazy, very excellent greyhound. Currently I am an opera singer, but I'm in the process of a career change into counselling and psychotherapy.

On 5th October 2019, I bounded (well, trundled - I very rarely bound) downstairs, pee-covered stick in hand and ceremoniously announced to my husband: "Well, it looks like we're going to have a baby then..."

5 weeks pregnant.

This is a story about miscarriage, and the way we talk about it (spoilers: it needs to change).

Like most women, I think, I was brought up on the idea that I must do *everything in my power* to avoid getting pregnant until I was "ready" (what does that even mean?) Such is the way our society demonises young mothers - but that's another story. I lived in fear of The Late Period. Every time I called my mother from uni with a life update of some sort, the first thing she'd say was "oh God you're not pregnant are you?". As a result, I'd been on the pill pretty much non stop since I was 17. I was 35 when we started trying for a baby, and friends and family fell over each other to tell me that it might take a while to conceive because I was "getting on a bit" and because it would take a while for 20 years of pill hormones to clear out. There was also my own awareness that, having hormonally blocked the option for so long, I had absolutely no idea whether I was able to have children at all. We were over the moon, then, to get pregnant very quickly. Not only were we fertile (phew!), but apparently impressively so (go us!) We had triumphed over the adversities of age and synthetic hormones and we were going to be parents.

6 weeks pregnant.

I was overjoyed to have very few symptoms. I wasn't really nauseous, apart from when I didn't eat enough (not a problem I normally have). I had sore boobs but nothing to write home about. Mainly, I couldn't sleep. I love sleep. However, despite this, I made peace with my lot and decided I could just about deal with it. I wanted to tell a few close friends, which I did, although the decision of who to tell carries so much weight. As well as not really trusting a test result that comes from you peeing on a stick you bought in your local Co-Op, it is apparently just Not The Done Thing to tell people before your 12-week scan. One of the reasons for this is "just in case"; the unspoken end of that sentence is of course "...you have a miscarriage". But nobody says that bit, so nobody really engages with the possibility of it happening.

This is the first problem, and it's a big one. We are, as a society, increasingly disinclined to be at peace with the fact that life is sometimes uncomfortable and hard (see my thoughts on mindfulness later on). As a result, we slip further and further away from being able to process that which is difficult, choosing instead to ignore it until it's staring us in the face. This has the effect of making it even harder when we cannot ignore it any longer. Perhaps if we spoke more openly and less dramatically about miscarriage (to name just one example), women would be free to share their whole pregnancy journey with more people at an earlier stage, if they wished to. This would mean increased support networks in the event of miscarriage or other complications, as well as not having to hide the (sometimes debilitating) first trimester symptoms in the workplace. Instead of early pregnancy being "A Big Deal" that we don't talk about, it could be "Not A Big Deal" that we do.

8 weeks pregnant.

I was on tour with work in Newcastle, and one day, I woke up realising that I'd had the best night's sleep I could remember in weeks. I immediately knew that all was not well. I texted a few aforementioned inner circle friends with my concerns, but the responses were all along the same line: "Oh, I had days when I forgot I was pregnant!", "Some pregnancies are just really lucky with no symptoms!", "Don't worry, everything is absolutely fine!"

I had a midwife appointment in the diary a couple of weeks later, so I decided I would just press pause on the worry, continue as if I was pregnant, but not let myself get too excited about it. I thought I would explain my concerns to my midwife and perhaps have an early scan, or a heartbeat check. The midwife's response, however, echoed that of my friends: "Oh I wouldn't worry about it at all, symptoms come and go, it's probably all fine!" No possibility of a scan or a check-up unless I had something I could reasonably take to the Early Pregnancy Assessment Unit (pain, bleeding etc).

At this point, I began to doubt my own intuition.

This is the second problem. Why, in a world where people are trusted (expected?) to self-diagnose so many things, is the default position that pregnant women "are worrying about nothing"? Maybe some are unnecessarily concerned, but couldn't we learn to work more holistically with each person, ascertaining and understanding their individual experience before unilaterally writing their concerns off? Essentially, what we end up doing is making our women mistrust their own bodies and minds. Truly, that is Not OK; it is arguably a form of (albeit unintentional) gaslighting. Of course, it is important to note that, like most NHS staff, our midwives are stretched for time and resources. I also recognise that I am fortunate to live in an area of the country where it's normal to have the same midwife throughout pregnancy. My stance here is entirely idealistic, but it's as good a starting point as any, I think.

11 weeks pregnant.

One Sunday evening, I went for a wee and there was some blood. My first reaction was "ah, I knew it". However, almost immediately, I backtracked. Having been repeatedly told I was probably just worrying over nothing (albeit by very lovely, very well-meaning people), I convinced myself it was probably just a result of the particularly enthusiastic sex I'd had the night before. Also, the internet is full of "bleeding in the first trimester is normal, don't worry!" A Google search told me not to use my menstrual cup just in case it was a miscarriage, so I found an ancient sanitary towel and tried to forget about it.

Over the next day or two, there was more blood, so I booked an early scan at the EPAU. I was told that things didn't look great, but that there was "foetal matter" in there that was consistent with 4-5 weeks' growth. Was I sure of my dates?

At this point, I felt confident enough to self-diagnose a missed miscarriage. The foetus had obviously stopped growing shortly before that really great night's sleep a few weeks back, and my body was only now ready to do something about it. (NB a side note for those who have not had to wrangle with the confusion of pregnancy dating: due to the high variation in cycle lengths and wide ovulation windows, pregnancy is dated from the first day of your last period, which means, for those with a regular cycle, "5 weeks growth" roughly equates to "7 weeks pregnant".)

I was sent home with a variety of leaflets, but not a huge amount of practical advice, and told to wait and see what happened. I didn't have to wait that long. I started bleeding a lot more the following afternoon (I decided to have a glass of wine at that point) and the "main event" started that evening. I'd spent the day researching what I could expect and how to manage it and was lucky enough to have found a blog (just one) where the author's experience echoed what I felt I was going through:

You can scan the above QR code with your phone, which will take you to the website below:

https://medium.com/ask-me-about-my-uterus/there-will-be-blood-what-nobody-will-tell-you-about-miscarriage-dbfe205d1d5a.

Essentially, this author felt, it was simply a case of biology. It was not an overly emotional experience, although obviously that might come and go. The "results of conception" (or "pregnancy material" as she'd found it referred to) were simply that. Some people collect what comes out, I read elsewhere, but that wasn't the way this particular lady rolled, and neither did it seem the right approach for me. In fact, most of the other stuff on the internet seemed to actively not apply to me:

What I was told I would probably feel	What I actually felt
Guilt / like a failure	My body was just doing what it was designed to do when faced with a non-viable pregnancy
Grief / need to reflect	This was just an annoying roadblock - frustration at having to start again
Lack of interest in physical contact	Overwhelming desire to have sex with my husband again - for intimacy as much as (if not more than) to start trying again

This is the third problem, and why I am so keen to specifically share my story with others. If there's a taboo around talking about miscarriage (and there is), there seems to be an even bigger one about not feeling particularly emotional about it.

Don't get me wrong, it was bloody painful, incredibly tiring and relentless. The husband and dog just set up camp next to me on the bedroom floor and we rode it out together. But I didn't cry (apart from in pain - miscarriage gives you a handy heads up on what contractions are like) and I certainly didn't feel like I was losing a baby that demanded to be grieved. Whoever I spoke to, despite my protestations that actually I felt ok, the response was the same: "give it time, it'll probably hit you when you least expect it". Everywhere I looked, I was told that I wasn't doing this in the expected way. The only time I felt understood (by somebody who didn't previously know me) was when the nurse came to give me the leaflets in the "reflection room" at the EPAU. She pointed out a memorial box that I could leave a message in if I wanted to, but then said "although I get the impression that isn't really very you". I loved that nurse.

We have to remove the societal messaging that the only way of processing a miscarriage is through devastation and grief. Women must, of course, be free to grieve if it is right for them, but it is not 'one size fits all', which effectively tells every woman that they have to grieve, whether they feel they need to or not. Also, by telling women over and over again that it's "normal" to feel like a failure, we tell them that that's what they are. Can we not be bold enough to trust people to process these things in ways that make sense to them? I was not devastated, I was pissed off because I am a planner and I hate being made to rethink my plans (2020 lockdown is doing wonders for this, incidentally). The NHS webpage on miscarriage deals exclusively with grief, and what it might feel like. Nowhere does it say "it's also ok to be ok". Dayna Winter's blog (link above) was a saving grace, because it made me realise I wasn't weird for reacting in a different way.

14 weeks (not) pregnant.

My understanding from Dr Google was that you have to wait until the bleeding stops and you have a negative pregnancy test before you start having sex again to reduce the chances of infection. This test, tallying with NHS advice, should be taken no earlier than 3 weeks after you've miscarried. I am not a particularly patient person, and as already mentioned, I was not going to wait any longer than necessary before having sex again. In the end, I managed to wait for two weeks before I took a test, but by that point I felt normal and was confident of a negative result. It was positive. Back in the EPAU, I was told that the miscarriage was incomplete, and being asked my preferences for removing the remaining tissue.

This was the point where I lost it a bit. I vividly remember thinking "I can't even miscarry properly". Even if these thoughts were short lived, the frustration got stronger. Why wasn't it over yet? I wanted to start trying again *immediately* and the universe seemed to be saying no.

I told them I wanted to go down the surgical route - it is my general approach to similar decisions to rip off the band-aid and get it done. They consulted with the doctor and came back to say that unfortunately this was not a possibility after all - the remaining tissue was so small that the risk of surgery was disproportionately high. Instead, I was sent home with a small pill and some more leaflets. The pill, incidentally, is designed to kickstart the 'natural' miscarriage process. Despite my protestations that my body had already tried that method and it hadn't worked properly, I was told I had to do this first before they'd consider any other options. Then I was to wait another three weeks (did I mention that I'm not a patient person?) before doing another test.

I took the pill and settled in for a second evening of pain. Nothing happened. I felt vindicated in my assertion that it wouldn't work. At one point, I went for a wee and a tiny tiny bit of clotted blood was on the loo paper, but it seemed too small to be significant. The next day, I called the EPAU to let them know it hadn't worked, and to ask for another scan to see what they thought.

It turns out the EPAU doesn't offer this option: "we can't offer follow up scans to everybody having a miscarriage because there simply aren't enough hours in the day".

This is the fourth problem. There is a *huge* disconnect between how the medical profession approaches miscarriage, even internally, and how society deals with it. A woman facing her first miscarriage is simultaneously told - directly or indirectly - the following things:

1. Miscarriage isn't common enough to be spoken about openly (see also: "you're worrying over nothing")

2. There isn't any reliable data because miscarriages are more common than you think, and it's impossible to know how many late periods are actually miscarriages
3. Having 3 miscarriages is incredibly uncommon
4. You won't get any special treatment in the NHS until you've had 3 miscarriages because it's deemed too normal before that point

I think we can all see what's wrong with this combination of things, and it's really not a separate problem, it's a combination of the previous three. Firstly, we ignore the existence of miscarriage. Then we tell women that it probably won't happen to them, despite happening "more often than you think". When it does happen, we tell women it's ok to feel like a failure, but not ok to accept it as a thing that sometimes happens and move on. "Mixed messages" doesn't really cover it, does it?

15 weeks (not) pregnant.

I took my second post-miscarriage test within the week (I didn't even make it to two weeks this time). When you're trying for a baby, willing a pregnancy test to come back as negative is a strange experience. It's a bit like an episode of Deal or No Deal, where somebody has taken a deal and spends the rest of the episode desperately trying to find the £250,000 that they were so keen to avoid at the start. The mental whiplash is quite something. But here I was, two and half months after celebrating the existence of an extra little blue line, thoroughly relieved not to see even the suggestion of one. I finally felt like I could move on with my life.

Six months later...

As I type this, I am around 18 weeks pregnant, having conceived during my first ovulation since miscarriage. We are (hopefully) having twins. Nonidentical, which means I ovulated two eggs at the same time. I mentioned that I'm a planner, yes? Nice to know my body still has a sense of humour...

I told a friend a couple of days ago that I am grateful for my miscarriage. This might seem a strange thing to say, but bear with me. I mentioned earlier about society's decreasing ability to sit comfortably with the uncomfortable. I firmly believe that this has to change. One way of doing this is through mindfulness, which I found almost accidentally through practising yoga. My miscarriage gave me the opportunity to put everything I'd learnt into practice, and it has strengthened my ability to stay present, something for which I am increasingly grateful as I experience pregnancy for a second time. It is very easy to be swept along by planning your future life (marketing built on guilt-tripping is a particular highlight of impending parenthood) and if you've experienced one or more miscarriages in your past, it's equally easy to assume that every twinge is a precursor to another one. I have experienced both of these on more than one occasion, but each time there's a little voice in my head telling me that, whilst it's ok to think these things, perhaps it might also be good to sit quietly with my bump for five minutes to remind myself what it's all about...

There were a few main sources of support throughout this whole period, and on into this pregnancy. I am incredibly grateful for a husband who respects the decisions I make and feelings I have about my body without question, because, in his words, my opinion trumps his on such matters. I am (cautiously) grateful for the wealth of information on the internet about these things, and for the services that exist to support women who *do* feel that they want to grieve or hold memorials. Practically, I owe one particular friend a substantial amount of my sanity - she went through a very similar thing a few months before me, and can always be trusted to be a level-headed source of help and support. When I texted her to tell her I thought I was miscarrying, she told me that if it turned out I was, I'd need at least two packets of super absorbent Always, some painkillers and to cancel all my plans because I wouldn't be going far from the loo for some hours, and it would likely be a couple of weeks after The Main Event before I stopped bleeding. She also told me that the time between scans in any subsequent pregnancy would feel like a lifetime. She wasn't wrong.

There is an important point to make here, though. The support I received from that friend was only there for me to call on because she chose to be counter-cultural and share her experience with me *when she was going through it*. By doing so, she was sowing seeds of support that I didn't even know I was going to need. This, I think, is the key. Since telling people about my miscarriage, many friends have opened up to me about their historic experiences of it, and this obviously forms an important part of the support process, and one that I'm grateful for. But think about how much *more* support we'd be providing for each other by sharing these stories before we knew they were needed. Obviously there is a natural spectrum of openness, and I don't for one moment expect all women to suddenly start shouting about miscarriage from the rooftops, but I don't think that is the limiting factor. I think more women would be happy to talk openly about it if it were a thing that was openly talked about. A nice chicken and egg problem there.

One final thing to mention is the role played by home pregnancy tests, and our readiness to accept a positive result as a guarantee of future parenthood. The home test was championed as a way of giving women greater control over their bodies, and it certainly still serves that purpose, but the test has been developed over time to give earlier and earlier results, without giving the full context of these. The chance of miscarriage at 3 weeks pregnant is pretty high; 31% according to a journal article cited by Very Well Family:

You can scan the above QR code with your phone, which will take you to the website below:

https://www.verywellfamily.com/making-sense-of-miscarriage-statistics-2371721#miscarriage-rate-after-implantation

If we are to maintain this ability to find out so early, I think we need to be free to talk about pregnancy in the first trimester without anybody making the assumption that parenthood is guaranteed. This can only help the awareness and acceptance of miscarriage, which in turn makes it easier in some ways for those who experience it. To achieve this, I believe we have to gently, but firmly, challenge this assumption whenever we encounter it. I am sure I visibly winced when a work colleague of mine proudly announced that she was going to be a grandmother, a fact she knew because her daughter had just peed on a stick that morning and "was already 6 weeks!" I have thought about that moment a lot since, and the fact that I wanted to say something but I didn't know what or how. My own dad said the same thing when we told him about the twins - "I'm going to be a grandad", he said, with a slight lump in his throat. This time I was more prepared: "Yes, hopefully", I said, "but there's a way to go yet, and I'm taking it a day at a time".

Lottie

Lottie is yet to start her journey to motherhood, but the severe pains and sweats she gets with her periods suggest that her journey may not be straightforward. It will only be after the pandemic that she will find out.

Understanding yourself seems to be the 'in thing'? As a yoga teacher and someone who would appear to the suited and booted as a 'right hippy' I no doubt have used the phrase 'when we understand ourselves' or 'learning to understand yourselves' or even 'the process of understanding oneself'. The ridiculous and somewhat frustrating thing is, that our bodies are changing daily so will we ever really truly understand ourselves fully?

I was 11 when I was on the upstairs phone listening into my mother's conversation with my great aunt, which I often did- I was a snoop from day dot! I heard Mum say that my older sister has started her period, to which Auntie Patty replied "Poor Meghs". They carried on speaking about how god awful periods were and how they'd both been sick on several occasions just like my sister had just been. I sat on the toilet that evening eyeing up the 'lady products' that always sat in close proximity to the loo, tampons, sanitary towels, night sanitary towels, panty liners, a smorgasbord of women's 'equipment'. None of these I really knew much about, the only experience I'd ever had with these delights was my 5 year old self once thinking I could create some jazzy wall art while I was waiting for a poo to brew. I thought to myself, 'when I start my period I'll only bleed a very small amount, I won't need one of those nappy like things.

Fast forward 10 years and you would've found me sat on a toilet in Heathrow arrivals- a welcome party!- for Meghan who had spent the best part of six weeks in India. Welcome party? Not so much! My dad was there to meet her at the gate. My mother was propping up my sweaty body on a toilet, having just bought me a sarong and holiday t-shirt from a gift shop because I'd sweated through my clothes and vommed down my top. The Toilet attendant asking my Mum through the cubicle door if I needed a paramedic? "No thank you" My mother replied, Mum had dealt with this a good few times before, with me and herself.

The car journey should have been filled with chat of my sister's exciting expedition, instead, they had to listen to me groaning and growling all the way from Heathrow to my parents' house south East of the River.

That night I strapped a maxi, maxi sanitary towel to my big granny 'period pants' and looked at it like a comfy new mattress for my foof! Some people will never know the safety and security of giant pads and doubling up on pants to make sure the sanitary towel doesn't skid off in the night like it can't cope with the pressure of its job.

There have been times in my life I haven't felt womanly, I am fairly straight up and down with a flat chest and broad shoulders- I'd sometimes overthink my period and think it was nature's way of telling me 'I was just so god damn fertile' and that my baby-box was punishing me for not being up the duff. Unfortunately now, as I get increasingly older and the want for a family comes into my thoughts weekly, it fills me with a little more worry. Worry that I won't be able to procreate and the pain I go through is indeed scarring behind my uterus. Only a further MRI will confirm that, what they have confirmed is that my womb lies too close to my bowel, possibly why I get IBS like symptoms around my period, I believe this is why my toilet humour Is. On. Point!

Have you tried the Pill asked Barbara? Barbara was a Doctor I met at a Women's clinic in East London one Wednesday afternoon. She seemed kind of interested in my predicament of prolific monthly pain- more so than any other doctor I'd met before, seemed like Babs worked in the right place. She quizzed me about my past history of 'period management contraceptive'- I'd tried it all! The pills, the injection etc. She sold me the idea of the coil pretty well, her Radio 4 tones and her middle aged, almost artsy appearance (unusual for a doctor I thought) lulled me into a 'safe zone'.

I was booked in the following Saturday. Barbara wasn't going to be inserting the coil; it would be her colleague. That Saturday I rocked up to the clinic having just knocked back a couple of ibuprofen- recommended to do by a friend, the doctor who sat before me didn't quite have Barbera tones, she was a little abrasive and wasn't fussed that I appeared a bit nervous. I asked her if it hurt? She said it wouldn't be comfortable. 'Why would it?' I thought after feeling daft for asking such a question. It's a bit of metal/plastic being pushed up and in! I followed her into a little room, the classic half-bed-chair with foot holders sat in the middle white cube like room. The nurse took my hand as I spread my legs, I could tell I was squeezing her hand a little harder than she'd anticipated I would.

The doctor was right, it wasn't comfortable! It was like Phil Taylor had thrown a winning dart straight into my cervix, but It was quick and stabby and like that it was done. The doctor left the room- I pulled on my clothes and the nurse went to get me some water. I went to leave, 30 seconds from when the nurse left and me getting up to go to the door, I felt the room spin on its head and my body rise with searing heat. The heat that I experience when I have a bad monthly episode, and within seconds I found myself back on the bed. Nurses rushing into the room and a nice 'nurse man' called Simon fanning my face, I promptly vomited. I heard a face say south of my belly button that they were keeping my dignity. Dignity? I wasn't fussed, you'd put in there lady, you fish the thing out! I could see the panic on her face as she tried to pluck out the bit of plastic that I can only describe looking a lot like a fishing hook. Apparently, I was going into shock. Going into Shock? What? No! this is just what happens each month, instead this time it had been manually triggered... weird! However, because I'd passed out they'd given me a shot of adrenalin (fun stuff) and hooked me up to a drip and a heart monitor. There are 2 things that happen that are visually a little 'off putting?' when I have an 'episode' I sweat! When I say I sweat, I've been known to slide off a toilet and drip through my clothes. If I close my eyes I can see the beads of sweat dripping into my pants as I lean forward clutching at my stomach. The second thing that happens is my heart rate plummets, this is something I only discovered during the coil incident. I wouldn't mind betting it's happened every time I've had an episode.

The turning point was last summer, I haven't been one to track or log my periods- I took the road of: 'if I don't know it's coming, I don't have to dread it!' That's the wrong road, it's a road that once took me down being in the back of a Croatian ambulance having just passed out on a ferry boat in the middle of a national park. It wasn't ideal! £140 later, my ID was released from the hospital having laid in the chaotic trolley bay for 2 hours and refusing an internal examination from a man who couldn't help looking a lot like Hannibal Lector.

It had reached its peak, I had to go and deal with this and speak to someone about what was going on, I have now been referred although understandably things are a little postponed because of the current pandemic.

I found a way of managing and planning for my period a little better, an app called Clue has been brilliantly helpful, even though 2 days before I'm due on I get a notification that says 'it's on its way' I feel the notification should come with jaws music... I now understand that ibuprofen (for me) makes me feel worse and that it's paracetamol that will help bring my temperature down, CBD oil is also another great discovery. And being open, with colleagues and friends. If I can't go into work- I shouldn't, if I can't go for dinner because I've spent most of the day in the bath I should just stay on the sofa with a hot water bottle! I've had a few months now where I haven't vomited or been writhing in the bath like a whale with the plague. I do of course worry as to what they might find when I do eventually get an MRI but for now taking as much control as I have the power to do is all that I can do, and it's better than doing nothing. Knowledge really is power, the more you can know about the little things really is helpful. Yes our bodies change daily but not shutting out, not being ashamed, doing some sensible research makes understanding this ever-changing system that is our body a little easier to manage.

Louisa

*Louisa has experienced a Termination for Medical Reasons (TFMR)
when her son Toby developed abnormalities. She has found much
support in the ARC support group, her husband, and her dog.*

      I am Louisa. I am 31 years old. All I've ever really
wanted is a nice guy, a dog and a baby. I have been married
to the nice guy for 6 years, 2 years ago I finally persuaded
him to get a dog. We had tried for over two years to get
pregnant; we were just about to go down the IVF route,
when in July 2019 we found out I was pregnant. We
couldn't believe it, how amazing, I was so worried
something would happen though. I only told my mum. We
went for our 12-week scan and everything looked fine, that
evening I told friends and they were so excited. After
hearing the heartbeat at the 16-week appointment I started
to think about the future and told people at work.

      The 20-week scan was actually at 21 weeks and it
was on my husband's birthday what a great birthday
present this was going to be. We had decided not to find
out the gender. We naively thought everything would be
fine and we would get to see our baby again. The
sonographer pointed out the organs and limbs but then she
said she couldn't see a part of the brain and went to get
someone else to look. This person agreed and we had to go
into another room, our worlds came crashing down. We
had to go to a specialist hospital the next day. I cried all the

way to the appointment; I couldn't believe this was happening. They did a very long scan; I couldn't watch but my husband did. Afterwards, they told us that there were a few problems with the brain and all the long bones were short. We were given 3 options: say goodbye now, have tests and then decide or have no tests and continue. We didn't know what to do, we said we'd go away and think.

Unfortunately, I felt quite negative and detached from the baby, I was thinking 'why us?'. But my husband was thinking positively as always. We went away for a few days which were already booked, it was very odd we were in a bubble away from reality. We had to decide what we were going to do which was so hard as the baby was inside me.

We decided to have more tests to find out more but I was anxious I had to go through these. The first one was an amniocentesis, they had to stick a big needle in to take some fluid from around the baby. The second was an MRI, I had to hold my breath twice which was hard. I turned into robot mummy getting through the procedures. Waiting for the results was such a difficult time, I didn't want to see anyone until we knew what we were going to do. I did a lot of colouring in this time. I was now 23 weeks pregnant and we had to make our decision by 24 weeks.

Results day, I think I already knew we would have to say goodbye but my husband was still hoping for the best. When they started listing all the abnormalities, I knew it would be too cruel to bring the baby into the world. We had to decide to have a TFMR (termination for medical reasons) The next day we had to go back so they could inject the heart so the baby wasn't born alive. This didn't really hit me; it was like it was happening to someone else. We found out it was a boy and called him Toby, a name we had thought about for years. I had to take a tablet to prepare for the birth and then go to hospital two days later. We went into hospital on the 24th November and the induction started. By the next morning, I was in a lot of pain and had to have some morphine. Toby was born sleeping at 10.44 on the 25th November. I felt disgusting and didn't want to meet him feeling like that, I had a shower and then a rest. When the lovely midwife bought him in, we couldn't believe his beautiful fingers and toes and his cute face. The midwife had taken pictures, measurements and hand and foot prints, He weighed 1 pound 5 oz. When we left that evening, we got to the lift at the same time as new parents with their baby in a car seat, we just had his memory box which was so sad.

The first few days were awful as I couldn't sleep and was so upset that Toby wasn't here. This was the saddest week of my life, I couldn't imagine my husband going back to work, me going back to work or ever being happy again. I have never cried so much, how can life be so cruel and how could anyone possibly understand what we have gone through. We decided to bury Toby at a cemetery close to our home. We couldn't have his funeral until 23rd December because we had to wait for him to have his post mortem, but we were glad we would know where he was at Christmas. Choosing poems for the service was so sad as it made it more real that he wasn't here. We had a grave side service with close family, the sun was shining and the birds were singing. The tears flowed but I realised this was a nice thing to do for him surrounded by love. I visited his grave every day for the first few months, I had to check everything was ok, this was all I could control for him now so I wanted it to be beautiful. We found out Toby had a deletion in the long arm of chromosome 13, this is what caused his abnormalities. Even though it's so sad we knew we had made the right decision.

Luckily my work was very understanding, the manager had a friend go through something similar. They sent a note around saying what had happened and that I do want to talk about Toby. January 20th was my first few hours back at work, they agreed I could slowly build my hours up. A couple of people mentioned Toby and said it was good to see me back but some people said nothing which was so sad. On Toby's due date we took our dog to the beach, we took the bear and book from his memory box with us. I wrote Toby in the sand and made a heart out of cream roses and put his bear in the middle. My husband made a star out of cream roses and read the book, I read a poem I had written to Toby. That evening we went to his grave and let off a balloon, at home, we lit a candle and both had a good cry. This was meant to be the day he came home and no one can really understand unless they have been through baby loss. One of my best friends had her baby a few weeks after Toby's due date, I couldn't talk about anything pregnancy related while she was pregnant, she was amazing and understood. The day her baby was born I had to read through Toby's diary and had a good cry, more because Toby isn't here rather than that her baby is.

Her baby is a little girl which I think helps. I left it a month before video calling her, on the video call she straight away said how sad it is that Toby isn't here with us and that her baby and Toby should be growing up together, this meant a lot.

Baby loss is the loneliest bubble to be in, people don't mention your baby because they think it will upset you but actually, I get more upset when they don't mention him. I feel like I won't be happy until I have another baby and I feel people will pity me until I have another baby. Six months on we now feel ready to start trying for Toby's brother or sister but we know this pregnancy will be filled with anxiety and stress. I still think about Toby every day and visit his grave several times a week, I love taking him fresh flowers. I have bad days and good days; at the moment I'm struggling with the jealousy and comparing, I have bought a positivity journal and hope this helps.

I am now so much more aware about baby loss and that very few have an easy ride to motherhood.

Things that have helped me
ARC charity which stands for antenatal results and choices.
When we had our scan and when making our decision, we received some very helpful booklets from ARC. After giving birth to Toby I emailed them to ask if I could go on their forum, I received their newsletter in the post. I read a mum's diary to her baby, it hit me so hard and I cried so much. It was the first thing I'd read that related to my situation, I read it over and over again. This inspired me to write a diary to Toby and I sent this to friends and

family. This helped me know that they knew what we had been through and how we were feeling. I still add to his diary now. The forum is for women who have had to make this awful decision. It helped me not feel so alone, being able to relate to people's posts. I met a lovely lady on there who had to say goodbye to her baby for similar reasons and similar timelines, we now message each other regularly, we understand each other.

My dog

I think he actually saved my life, I had to get up to take him for a nice walk. He was always there for cuddles.

Personalised Jewellery

For Christmas my husband got me a pendant with Toby's footprints and name on. I wear it every day and fiddle with it at work.

Books

'Saying goodbye' and 'The baby loss guide' by Zoe Clark-Coates were our bibles at the beginning, she has had five losses and has two living children.

'Ask me his name' by Elle Wright – Elles baby Teddy died at three days old, very emotional but I found it so relatable and it's lovely how she keeps the memory of her son going.

'The burden of choice' edited by Georgina Pearson is a collection of stories from parents facing a diagnosis of abnormalities during pregnancy. It is a very emotional read but makes you feel less alone.

Blogs

An unexpected family outing- This is a lady in America who has had a miscarriage, a still birth and now has a little girl. It's like she has taken the words from my head and again is just so relatable.

Feathering the empty nest- Elle Wright who wrote the book above has her own blog, she writes about her own experiences and also has a mum's voice blog series where mums share their baby loss stories.

And of course, my Husband who held me in the middle of the night, wiped away my tears and helped me through the hardest 6 months of my life.

Lucy

Meet Lucy, who shared laughter with her husband through the more uncomfortable moments of IVF.

I live in London with my husband, and I'm 35 years old. I've done a lot of different jobs, including working for myself, and more recently in tech startups. I'm currently half way through a masters course. We started seeking answers about why we couldn't conceive when I was 32 and he was 31. We had one fresh and one frozen embryo transfer on the NHS, and a third embryo transfer in a private clinic.

In writing my story, I can't help but reflect that I don't know if I would have found it useful in the midst of treatment. Strangely, rather than accounts of successful fertility procedures, I hunted for stories of people who had finished it without children. I wanted to know that it was possible to build a full and happy life afterwards, without a child. More than that, I wanted to know how you knew when to stop trying and how others had made that decision, and how they reflected on it in the years that followed. Back then, I found the tabloid stories of 'I conceived after 11 cycles of IVF' distressing, and now I find them exploitative. Was I supposed to sacrifice all and everything, to keep going until we were successful? Is that how it worked? The articles were written as if they were supposed to give you hope, but I felt hopeless in the face of them. I didn't think I could emotionally and physically commit to such a process, let alone financially, but how could I make a decision to stop? Clinics, waiting rooms and articles all focused on hope and success. I wanted to know what would happen without it.

Luckily for me, it never came to that. I side-stepped the pain of that decision. After our third embryo transfer, I became pregnant with twins, and they held on for 37 weeks + 5, then born in a July heatwave. I had only had one egg collection, with good results and a good number of frosties in the freezer. I responded well to the drugs, without many side effects. In IVF terms, I had certainly had a very smooth experience, but I had still said to my husband that if this third attempt didn't work, I needed a proper break. Not just the few weeks I'd asked for between attempts two and three, but some clear months, with no guarantee I'd return to the process. Even that was a difficult tussle. Should I bank some eggs in my last months before turning 35, to give us the freedom to forget about things for months, or even a year? Or were our frosties enough? This calculation of numbers, searching for certainty in percentages of success and failure, was constant.

I hadn't always known definitively that I wanted to be a mother. To aspire to quiet domesticity and family seemed less exciting in comparison to a desire to travel or to build a career, or somehow do something, but the adolescent desire to *do* something has faded comfortably into the distance. In my twenties, I hunted for accounts of women making decisions about whether to have children or not, with the same fervour I would later have for articles about not being able to have them at all. Again, I found them to be focussed on the happy ending of children, and lacking a happy ending of not. In other ways I felt there was no decision needed. To see my husband with children was to know he should be a father.

My husband and I had a quick and concrete diagnosis for our failure to conceive - another piece of infertility luck - and were soon on the path to IVF. I refused to go ahead before attending an adoption induction meeting, which left me feeling I certainly wasn't ready to commit to adoption or fostering. In fact, it made me feel far readier for IVF than I had felt before. While I might have been uncertain about a baby in theory in the years beforehand, the process of fertility treatment garnered a deep longing and many moments of desperate hope and desperate grief. I wonder if I had chosen to be child-free, if these moments of hope and grief would have descended on me similarly, but years later.

The middle Sunday of the two week wait was generally the moment of breakdown. Every couple of days in the lead up to the embryo transfer there would be a scan, a new drug, something that felt like progress or action, increasing in frequency until the transfer came. And then suddenly, you were cut loose. No analysis. No progress reports. Just you and a body and days that needed to pass. The first day or two would be full of hope and doom, the following days of denial and keeping it together, until a week in, when a full breakdown would ensue - snot and tears and despair. Followed by concern that the breakdown had been stressful, and stress could harm our chances. No hot bath, no yoga, no swimming, no wine, to relieve the stress.

After our first embryo transfer, we initially had a positive result. Three days later, when I was in a meeting, I noticed the cramps I'd had regularly were stronger than usual. My back was sore. I went to the toilet and my brain forgot. 'Oh, my period', it thought. A second passed. Then I remembered I wasn't supposed to be having a period.

At the early pregnancy unit the following morning, they wouldn't confirm a miscarriage, and wouldn't for several weeks. I needed to return multiple times for an internal scan before they'd call it, whilst being told to continue on my IVF drugs, knowing it was over, resentful of the futility of the hormones. At a follow-up appointment before starting the next round, a nurse passingly commented that if it happened again I'd need to collect the 'products of conception'. It was said so passingly and with no clarification that it took a little while for my brain to catch up. I noted it as a question to ask at the next appointment. What in god's name could the logistics be for that? How? In what? An uncomfortable doctor flushed when we asked him for guidance. He said at home, we didn't need to worry. At hospital, he said....He floundered...they'd use a..well, um...a. He didn't want to say. He barely whispered the words, 'sick bowl'.

Poor man, we found his discomfort quite funny. Like when we were sat in the clinic waiting room, thought the classical music on the radio was a bit depressing, and they announced it was the theme from Schlinder's List. Or when the first doctor to wield an internal probe at me proudly announced his name, the same name as my father-in-law. Moments of shared laughter at the absurdity of things helped us through.

We were also recording our experiences, and the mechanism of a regular interview or recording really helped us make room for talking about what we were thinking and what our experiences were. We were very reliant on each other, as we told very few people about treatment. We told my sibling and a very few close friends. Pub visits and off-loading, venting to those friends really helped, but so did limiting who we told. It was helpful that not all our social interactions involved 'how's it going' questions. I think sharing is hugely powerful and helpful, but not everyone has a right to the moment by moment updates on your medical treatment, and I often savoured our privacy. It meant when others announced their pregnancies to the group, I didn't have everyone looking to examine my reaction, or make a show of being especially congratulatory to smooth over discomfort.

It also meant that I avoided lots of platitudes that I'm hearing now. We've decided, currently, that we are done. Twins are enough for us. We can't bring ourselves to defrost and say goodbye to the frosties yet, which is yet another thing I'd like to hear the decision making stories about. But when I declare that we're having no more children, I'm given small smiles, and 'you never knows'. Even when I state that our diagnosis means that it's impossible for us to conceive naturally, people still want to suggest otherwise. I understand it. It feels like a positive thing to say, but I'd rather not sign up for those days of fraught and uncertain hopes again. Clarity has its own value.

A lot of the things that helped us aren't necessarily available to everyone. An understanding workplace and a job with flexibility and the ability to work from home. Taking an extra month out between cycles to have a proper break relies on you feeling you have time. For the cycle that worked, I cleared my schedule, so that after the embryo transfer all I needed to do was sit on the sofa and watch Line of Duty, and play meditation tracks on Spotify to calm me when I felt my feelings rise. I recommend a good TV police procedural - just the right level of distraction.

I worked on building an alternative life that could continue without children - I applied for courses that interested me, thought about possible travels, placed something in the future, not defined by fertility treatment. I also found it easier when I'd really come to terms with being in treatment, rather than denial. At the beginning, I tried to continue doing all the things I did before. When I slowed down, rested, took care, treatment felt easier to deal with. I logged into Instagram and periodically checked into some forums to feel comfort in reading about others' experiences and familiarity with the process. I listened to podcasts, 'IVFML' and 'Matt and Doree's Eggcellent Adventure'.

Each of our embryo transfers were given a name, and the second two were given a song. The second embryo transfer was named Yoshimi, so now when I hear the Flaming Lips' song, I can think about it. After the third I listened to Regina Spektor's Birdsong, so I thought about those lyrics a lot, about what might happen next; ' Out of the silence/ Might come the love song/ After the love song/ Might come the sunrise/ After the sunrise/ Might come the silence.'

Marlene

Marlene has only one ovary and little chance of natural conception, so she and her husband chose adoption, and now have grown from a family of 2 to a family of 11.

When I was 15 I was rushed into hospital. Apparently, I had a cyst on my right ovary. It was removed, I went back to school, took my exams, went to teacher training college, met my wonderful husband to be and secured a teaching position which I loved dearly. Then we decided to try for a family........After deciding it was the right time to start a family we gave up on Durex and hoped all would be well.

3 years later- no luck so after a few tests I went into hospital for a full investigation. When I came round I was told 'I'm sorry my dear but you must have known from a previous operation you have no right ovary and the left one is so damaged you would only have 2% chance of conceiving'

You can imagine how I felt- my world collapsed in a sentence.

As a primary school teacher, I'd dreamed of having my own children.

My husband was amazing. He was my support. I hated magazines, they all had baby features and I wouldn't watch ITV too many baby ads.

Then he tentatively suggested adoption. I had thought about it but men back in the 70's wanted their own and were not usually open to the idea. Bless him we discussed it for about 2 minutes then contacted an adoption agency. This will be perfect- we are both regular church attendees so applied to The C of E adoption society and waited and waited...

After 2 months they replied suggesting we try our local council adoption society which we had done but they were not in a position to take it forward. We wrote again to the Church of England this time to the Children' Society. They were quite helpful but suggested we wait 6 months and apply again as I 'may fall pregnant'!

We waited exactly 6 months and wrote again. After another 3 months we had a reply!!! Yes, we were to be put on their register subject to police, background, immediate family and home situation reports. Would you believe it after 2 weeks of being accepted by the Children's society our local council said they had opened an adoption office!

Well, we were visited by some lovely people who wanted to know literally everything about us. Parental background, police records, our income all valid points but I just wanted my baby!!

Finally, we were assigned an adoption officer- she was so lovely. The Sunday before we were due to sign official papers for the adoption process to go ahead, I passed out in church with acute pain and was rushed to hospital where I was diagnosed with acute gallstones!

Naturally, we informed our adoption officer we couldn't sign as I was in hospital whereupon the agency contacted us to say the adoption couldn't proceed as I was likely to have a recurrence of the gallstones! You can imagine after coming so far to meet another hurdle.

I burst into tears and was still crying when the doctor came to see me to say I could be discharged. That set me off again- he wanted to know what was wrong and I told him the whole story. 'Right,' he said, ' I'll take them out in the morning.'

Whilst I was still in hospital recovering, the adoption office came with the official forms for my husband and I to sign.

'Congratulations, Mr and Mrs Evans you can now consider yourselves pregnant- in about 9 months you should be holding your baby!' In about 9 months we'll be holding our baby!

I returned to teaching and life continued - Christmas holiday, Easter holiday, Summer holiday- time seemed to crawl.

We were tentatively buying bits and pieces for our new arrival- nothing blue, nothing pink.

The summer holidays were over and I started a new term. As I was writing lesson plans the phone rang. 'Bother, someone would phone now!'

'Mrs Evans?' The voice was our social worker- I held my breath. 'Your baby is waiting for you, you may collect her next week!' A little girl! I burst into tears!

She asked me to put the phone down and contact Norman - she would phone back within the hour. Norman was beside me - as he has always been - within 15 minutes!

We were given basic details none of which I can remember but the following week we were to collect our little girl.

Panic buy time!!! Nappies, bottles, formula, steriliser and clothes (some pink)

The wonderful day arrived. We met our lovely social worker and together we went to a cosy terraced house in Swansea. There we met the adoption officer and a fantastic foster mum.

In an enormous pram surrounded by pillows was our beautiful, 3-week old baby daughter. I stroked her tiny hand with my index finger - she held on so tightly to my finger and looked straight at me - it was a bond never broken.

After a few formalities, we thanked her foster mother for taking care of her for us and along with half a tin of her current formula and a bottle, we took our baby home!

Our lives had changed forever.

The next hurdle was the 6 months wait before the official signing in court of the adoption papers - always at the back of my mind. But time flew by and all official papers were signed - she was our baby at last!

Time passed so quickly, she grew to be a beautiful, outgoing, very loved little girl.

When she was 2 she handed me a Mothercare catalogue I'd be reading.

'Mummy, I want him for a brother'

I couldn't believe it! She had actually put in motion the hope of a second adoption.

We were approved in the December and the following July our darling daughter held her 2-week old baby brother. He was the exact replica of the baby in the Mothercare catalogue!

For years she would tell friends and neighbours' I chose my brother from a catalogue!'

So that is our story- how 2 people became a family of 4. Now with a son-in- law and a daughter-in-law and beautiful grandchildren the 2 have become 11.

Goodness knows what the future may bring. We have been so blessed!

Naomi

Naomi silently suffered from Endometriosis for many years before it was diagnosed. She now talks confidently about the condition with her husband and those around her.

I'm Naomi, a 33 year old English teacher from the home counties. I have 2 little dogs, who are my babies and a wonderful husband. We are hoping that soon we will have a small person to add to our family.

My Mum always had the most awful periods and PMT – I used to worry that I would be the same. A worry that sadly turned out to be the case. She struggled for years to get pregnant with me, and she wasn't able to have any more. She got cervical cancer when I was fairly young, and although she survived, it meant no more children for her (although she was elated to wave goodbye to her periods.)

Mine started when I was 10 – I was on a school trip and was pretty convinced that I was going to die under a large (and rather terrifying) waxwork of Henry VIII. My teacher informed me that I was not going to die, but I was going to have to endure this monthly visit for approximately the next 40 years. Not the answer I was hoping for...

Fast forward to my teenage years and it was a time of bleeding through many lovely outfits, having to cancel plans and spending a lot of time doubled up on the floor crying and wishing I had been born without a womb. After much convincing, my Mum finally agreed to let me try the pill (she was terrified I was going to start having an 'adult' relationship with my older boyfriend who was at university...as though this couldn't happen unless I was on the pill.) And it worked, for a while. My periods were hardly a walk in the park, but they weren't quite as horrendous (although the lovely boyfriend did have to change his sheets and wash my clothes more than once) and I felt pretty normal. I would have pain flare ups every now and then and my emotions were always a bit unpredictable (sorry lovely boyfriend), but I felt ok. This pretty much stayed the same until my late 20s.

It was when I was about 27, in 2013, that things started to get much, much worse. I don't know if it was just timing, or the stress, but my womb started playing up all of the time. Not just that dreaded week of the month, but all the time. I had recently moved away with my boyfriend (not the same lovely boyfriend) to a completely new city. I had left behind a job I loved, my friends and family and my health started to suffer. Suddenly I was having cramps on any given day, shooting pains in my abdomen and sex was so incredibly painful at times that it became something I would dread. Some days my stomach would be fine; other days I looked as though I was 8 months pregnant (my up and down weight was something my partner loved to pick at). I had no idea what it was, but I knew it wasn't ok. I tried to talk to my partner about it; he was dismissive and told me it was all in my head. He was pretty angry about the sex situation and didn't take my pain seriously at all. A few months later we got married and when I had a flare up on our honeymoon it was the beginning of the end for me...He shouted and said some things that didn't help, but he also seemed to manage to convince me that I was exaggerating the pain and so I didn't seek help for myself. I was back to the teenage girl who accepted that bad periods were part of life and that was that. I started working part time as I hoped that might ease the burden – I was convinced people thought I was lazy and pathetic.

In 2015, my marriage was in tatters (a story for another time) and I was at my lowest. I moved back to the safety net of my friends, and along with my parents, they helped me rebuild myself. My self-esteem was on the ground and my pain had just become part of life for me. I lived on painkillers, hot water bottles and pretending I was fine. I think I was embarrassed, as though I was unable to cope with something that was 'normal' for other women. Day to day tasks such as walking the dog or taking out the rubbish would cause me so much pain, I began to hide myself away. I was terrified of all men; pretty sure I would never be able to have sex again and was ready to accept this as my new life. Luckily, my Mum and my friends were not going to allow me to do this. It took hundreds of appointments, internal and external ultrasounds, hormone pills, failed painkillers, doctors telling me 'no' and being sent home from work before one doctor took me seriously.

So finally, in 2017, I underwent investigative surgery. When I came round, the surgeon told me that the flesh below my belly button was gangrenous and if it had been left for much longer, I could have got septicaemia and died. They had taken a lot away, he said, and part of one of my ovaries had paid the price. They had managed to just avoid my womb, but it had been very nasty in there and he was concerned. They biopsied what they had taken and told me it was endometriosis. I had some idea of what this was, but not in any real depth (I think it is a crime how underplayed and underrepresented this illness is). As he talked, I found myself worrying more and more...he told me there was no cure, that I could have several more flare ups, that it can cause infertility...not things you want to hear when you are 30 and newly divorced.

So here we are in 2020. A month after my surgery in 2017 (and a month of my wonderful Mum looking after me and getting me back on my feet) I met my now husband. I had the courage to be honest with him from the get-go about my condition and how it impacts my life. Sadly, the surgery didn't really work, and I live on painkillers, and in constant pain. My endo belly flare ups are still the bane of my life – I spent most of our honeymoon looking pregnant (although we still had the most incredible time) – but he is supportive, patient and completely accepting. He has read up on it and always looks after me when I need it. I have found support in online communities; I genuinely had no idea how many women live with this illness. I read a lot about it and find that so many women are willing to share. Once you realise you are not alone, it helps you quantify and embrace your own situation. I speak about it openly with my friends, no longer ashamed or embarrassed about what I am living with. Recently, reading 'Conversations with Friends', by Sally Rooney, the protagonist was diagnosed with endometriosis. It was so empowering to read this and made me realise that this is not something to hide away or hide behind. I still hate my 'endo belly', but I am more comfortable that it is part of who I am.

My mother was my greatest support, always validating what I felt, comforting me when it was needed and helping me pull myself together when that was needed too. Having suffered so much herself, she always understood. I lost her 18 months ago and the grief pulled me back down again, but with the support of my incredible GP, friends and husband, I have started to climb my way back up. Around the same time, I stopped taking my pill and my husband and I decided to start trying for a family. I had basically been told that there were no other real options for me but a hysterectomy and so we decided that it might be time to have a family. We've decided to just have the one child and then I will have the surgery to hopefully stop my endo for good.

We haven't had any luck yet and have just started investigative tests at the fertility clinic. I feel excited, a little scared but quietly confident that we will be parents – just might take a while to get there. IVF – I'm ready for you.

Instagram @mrstbythesea

Nicole

Nicole uses spiritual practice and sketching to help soothe herself after a miscarriage. I met her via Twitter, but soon after, she left the social media platform. Wherever you are, Nicole, I wish you love.

My name is Nicole and I live in the North East, UK. My passions are connecting with nature, spiritual growth and learning how to navigate this rather difficult world via alternate methods of spiritual practice and conscious living rituals.

After being diagnosed with PCOS last year my world fell apart, I felt like grief was coming over me at the thought at not being able to conceive. My partner and I had been using the cycle method as a contraception method for the last 6 years of our 9-year relationship (not 100% safe that's a given) but we would usually plan to make love either just before or after my menstruation and never in my fertile window and be careful with ejaculation just in case. It had dawned on me that in that time of roughly following this method that we had never fell pregnant even when 'happy accidents' had happened and they had happened a fair few times, I knew then that my PCOS had a part to play in this, I just had a very late diagnosis after many years of occasional painful sex and unusual hormonal changes resulting in very bad mood swings and depressive episodes.

However in Oct 2019 my partner and I decided we were no longer going to follow the cycle method and let nature take its course, we felt that we were ready to start a family, with no real dates in mind of when we wanted a baby to come along, we were letting baby decide for us. It took us only 2 fertile windows to realise that I was late on my period and we then discovered I was pregnant with our very first baby. We were legit over the moon albeit very nervous. The first scan went amazingly and the buzz around baby and me and my partner was amazing, friends and family were ecstatic for us and we started planning the baby's room. We spent roughly £900 on baby furnishings, clothes, and even started to bulk on items like baby shampoo and nappies.

However, upon reflection it was when I reached 17 weeks pregnant that I started to feel a little underwhelmed by the whole thing and I couldn't come to terms with buying any more baby items, my moods were changing rapidly and I noticed my morning sickness had subsided rapidly. I felt like my normal self but it was like everything had a grey haze, I started to get extreme pain in my lower right side; that pain was usually associated with PCOS and it slipped past the midwife as just pregnancy pain. Two weeks later I had two dizzy spells followed by a collapse in Tesco. I was rushed to the Pregnancy assessment unit at my local hospital and unfortunately, there was no heartbeat on the doppler and no heartbeat on the scan. Our world ended there and then. We were in the midst of the coronavirus hype and we had lost our baby on 15.02.2020, not knowing where our future or where the country was headed.

On 17.02.2020 at 22.05pm we delivered our angel baby after 8 hours of induced labour and roughly 1 hour of intense contractions. She was no bigger than the sizer of my flattered hand, she was in perfect form and she was perfect. We named her Elsie Lea (Elsie after my Great Aunt and Lea after my partner's middle name 'Lee' but we added an 'A' on the end to make it unique and girly to Elsie) ... we then left home the next morning after a consultation and many bloods later with no baby. We were absolutely devastated. So far my mam has been my rock though this and because she lives opposite to us, she visited every day buying us shopping and making us coffee etc. My body took roughly 4 full weeks to heal, which included 3 and a half weeks of bleeding, severe migraines, inability to eat and bad episodes of shame and guilt.

The thing that got me through and the thing that is still getting me through is forcing myself out of bed on a morning and being with my partner. Unfortunately, my bereavement sessions have been postponed due to coronavirus and I can no longer see family members due to lockdown so I am having to distract myself as much as I can with walks and sketching until I can see my family again. It is a very challenging time. But I will get through this just like all other bereaved parents.

Rebekah

*Rebekah wanted to start a family young but discovered she had
PCOS. Through a lifestyle change, a loss of weight and that magic
word Luck, she now has 3 wonderful children.*

I'm Rebekah. I'm 35 years old. I'm a wife, a teacher,
a daughter, a friend and a mother.

I married young; graduated Uni and having a
wedding in the same week sort of young. In my naïveté I
thought that we'd soon have a small person running
around the place because obviously all we had to do to get
pregnant was have un- protected sex right? I mean that's
what we're taught all throughout high school, you have sex
you will have a baby. Taught to a point that the lack of
understanding of how my own body worked at that point
in time was frankly embarrassing.

But it didn't happen.

My cycle had always been irregular and every time
it didn't appear in a 'normal' time frame my excitement
would mount. I'd start spotting every symptom going –
that was definitely a twinge of morning sickness, maybe
my want for pancakes was actually a craving. Were my
boobs feeling bigger and achey?

This went on for just over a year. Each time the
stick told me no my heart would start to feel a little bit
heavier and the doubts began to leak in. So I tried the
ovulation sticks and nothing. No smiley faces for me. I peed

on one of those buggers every day for over two months and nothing. This finally got me to go to the doctors. I hated doing this. It felt like I was letting the side down by admitting there was something wrong and that I was showing my weakness.

They started investigating with blood tests and an external ultrasound. Blood tests that had to happen on certain days of my cycle, a cycle that just wasn't happening. Eventually, the tests lead to my diagnosis of Polycystic Ovary Syndrome; I had off the chart levels of testosterone and lots of lovely scarring on my ovaries. This info was delivered to me by a lovely Socorro who shared her own fatality issues with me but ended with a kindly meant but bluntly given conclusion of how she'd never seen scarring this bad and not to get my hopes up that I'd ever get pregnant naturally.

Crushed isn't really the right word for it. Devastated? Heartbroken? A failure? How do you put into words having the rug pulled out from under you like that? The impact on your mental health of being told, what you have always seen as a fundamental part of being a woman, is unlikely to happen for you? Failure is what I felt and how I saw myself.

The rest of the appointment was a blur but I do remember managing to hold the tears back long enough to walk the short distance from the surgery to my husband's shop, locking the door behind me and just crumpling into gasping sobs as I tried to explain it all. Simon was absolutely my rock through all of this. He held me together physically and metaphorically as I shattered into a million little pieces. He brought in the loving support and reinforcement of my parents who drove the three hours journey from theirs to ours in breakneck speed to wrap me in their loving embrace.

The next steps were meant to be appointments with the specialist to look at IVF and if that was a viable option for us. But we never got that far. Somehow, going against all the odds, I had fallen pregnant naturally with no intervention other than losing weight. Carrying excess weight when you have PCOS can increase symptoms- I wasn't even out of a healthy BMI but the extra half a stone clearly was making a big difference. We were blessed with our eldest, a beautiful girl, Lyla.

She would then, five years later; after more investigation from a specialist; a lifestyle change; a number years trying and the use of advice from Chinese medicine be joined by her beautiful brother Dexter and 22 months after that by our youngest, Freddy.

Now, looking back over all the tears and heartbreak I went through I sometimes feel rather foolish and that maybe my story doesn't have a place amongst those of miscarriages and fertility treatment that never resulted in a baby. But, I wanted to share to give others hope. In my darkest moments, I never believed I'd be a mother of one let alone three. But there they are our mini humans who are all a gorgeous combination of the two of us.

Sera

Sera has wanted to be a midwife since she was a child. A few years into the career, she knew that there was an area she wanted to specialise in, and since then, she has spent her time supporting grieving families in her role as a bereavement midwife.

When you tell someone you're a midwife the response is always 'that must be a lovely job'. When I say I am a bereavement midwife the response is very different. They don't know how to react and that's because we live in a society that's uncomfortable talking about grief and heartache.

When I became a midwife 13 years ago, I always knew I wanted to be a community midwife and specialise in an area. For me, midwifery was about building relationships with women and their families, building trust and understanding their journey. Community midwifery meant I could build these relationships throughout the whole pregnancy not just in 1 shift where you look after a woman in labour. I think every midwife knows quite quickly which area they want to work in, it is definitely a calling and a vocation. I specialised as a bereavement midwife 5 years ago, I was always interested in the role which I realise sounds morbid to some. I just wanted to support these families in any way I could.

The role of a bereavement midwife varies across the country as does the support offered to bereaved families. This is one of the things that I'm most passionate about. I think it is totally unacceptable that one woman will get more support than another depending on where she lives. Unfortunately, the postcode lottery of the NHS affects many different fields.

I am very fortunate to work in a hospital trust that values the bereavement service and encourages us to do our job well. As a community bereavement midwife, I care for families after they have come home from the hospital. These families may have lost a baby from 12 weeks pregnant to full term or neonatally. I work with a wonderful team of bereavement midwives that look after these families during the labour and birth, help them make memories and spend time with their baby. I offer support visits and phone calls as often as needed for 3 months following the birth. How much support is given is led by the families and taken at their pace.

During these visits, I listen; I listen to their story, I listen to their grief, I listen to their questions, I listen to their anger, I listen to their guilt and blame. Then I ask; I ask about their baby, I ask his/her name, I ask to see photos/hand and footprints if they would like to share, I ask about their memories made in such a short time and I ask how I can help. Everything I know and do I have learnt from the families I have supported. Everyone grieves in such different ways but yet they all want to talk and remember their babies, they all feel guilty and blame themselves and they always ask if they are normal. It's amazing how as humans we can even question if we are grieving correctly?

I'm not sure if you can ever make the unimaginable pain of losing a baby any better for someone but I like to think knowing someone is there makes a difference. The most important thing that anyone can do is acknowledge their baby, make sure you ask his/her name and give the person as much time as they need to talk about their baby. They may tell you the same thing over and over but every time they do it is therapy and you are helping them through their grief.

Often people ask me how I can do my job and don't I find it depressing? I feel massively privileged to be let into a family's home during the worst time in their life, that they welcome a stranger in and share their most raw or painful thoughts and tell me about their lives. The relationships I build will never be forgotten, the families will always be special and thought of often. I have learnt so much from them and I have been shaped by them. When I leave their homes, I am in awe of them and the incredible strength they have.

The best part of my job is that I get to caseload these women throughout their next rainbow pregnancy as their midwife. I get to be part of this most incredible journey, to reassure them, help ease their anxiety and encourage their joy. Then when they bring their baby home I get to watch them build the life they had previously imagined, to make those memories they dreamt of whilst honouring the memory of their angel baby. What could be more wonderful than that?

Shareena

Shareena, diagnosed with PCOS, knew she'd have difficulties in having children, but this didn't stop her determination. Shareena speaks from the heart, has been through a lot, and has a good knowledge of the technical vocabulary that comes with the territory.

So I was diagnosed with polycystic ovaries at the age of 21, when I went to the doctor to ask why I only had a period once a year!! I was told then I would probably have trouble having kids! Then I met Fred who has a spinal cord injury (T12-L1-L2, crush), because of this he doesn't ejaculate! After being together 3 years I was diagnosed with abnormal cells, thankfully no cancer, but was told maybe to consider having kids soon, so we started trying.

After 3 years, no luck unsurprisingly, and through referrals, we ended up at Midlands Fertility Clinic for IVF. After consultation, they decided to do ICSI, where they surgically remove sperm and inject it into the egg directly. However as I didn't have periods, they had to stimulate me to have periods before I could start a cycle.

Once our first cycle began, I didn't react to the drugs, so they kept upping the levels of hormones, but as the levels were so high, I produced 60 to 70 follicles, so the eggs were really poor quality, so they fertilised them, but then I hyperstimulated so they froze them. On defrosting they shattered so we got nothing from it.

The next round went kind of the same way, but they put them back in, I hyper stimulated and was on bed rest for two weeks.

The third round again went the same way, however, the hyperstimulation was so bad that I vomited for about three days straight, Fred drove me to A and E, I was going in and out of consciousness with the pain, A&E left me in the waiting room for about for about 4 hours I was in so much pain I begged Fred to take me home which he eventually agreed to. He took me to the clinic the next day, where they immediately put me on a drip to rehydrate me and blue lighted me to hospital. Unsurprisingly I didn't get pregnant.

After that, they refused to let me do IVF as it was too dangerous!!

We tried a couple of rounds of donor IUI, but because of my polycystic ovaries I couldn't ovulate so then we looked at adoption.

When contacting the adoption agency I was told off quite severely for calling myself half-caste and didn't I know that was racist!! Then we stayed on the list for 2 years until they finally told us that as our County didn't have any mixed-race kids we wouldn't be adopting anytime soon. So we went to Thailand to stay with family and decompress, we volunteered in orphanages there.

Finally, on arrival back, we contacted the fertility clinic and asked what we could do, they suggested donor embryos, where embryos from other couples IVF rounds are donated to couples. The list was about 5 years and growing, so we added ourselves to the end. To go on the list you have all sorts of blood tests and I came out with being positive for a harmless virus that lives in about 10% of the population. Luckily for us, the couple donating also had this virus and as you can only then donate to virus-positive people, as I was the only person with it, we moved from the end of the list to the front.

On first trying, my womb lining wouldn't form properly, so the attempt was abandoned before the embryos were defrosted, the second attempt was a success in forming the lining and so they defrosted all four donated embryos, unfortunately, they weren't that great, two shattered, one split and one wasn't growing as it should, they implanted two and we were put on a course of drugs.

Two weeks later we had a pregnancy scan and YAY YAY YAY!

Couple weeks later at work I stood up to find I was covered in blood, went to A and E and had a scan to show that all of my womb lining had ripped away except the bit where Zach was attached, so was put on bed rest and told not to hope, but 12 weeks later the scan showed everything progressing well. Everything was easy and fine until birth, where Zach tried to strangle himself with his cord, but one happy baby boy born safe and well.

Not ever really tried for another, though I really long to, Zach has "brothers" from his original round of IVF who are 10+ years older than him.

Sophie

Sophie felt silly flagging symptoms of preeclampsia but her encounter with an amazing midwife saved the day and led to her son being induced several weeks early.

My name is Sophie and I am a 32 (how did I get to be 32?!) year old mum of one, a very "active" two-year-old called Atticus. When I'm not chasing a partially wild toddler around, I'm a full-time English teacher and moved back to Guernsey, nine years ago.

"Oh, aren't you just glowing", is a statement nobody ever greeted a soon to be mum with preeclampsia with! One of the many joyful symptoms of preeclampsia is excessive swelling (and I mean, EXCESSIVE!), so by my seventh month of pregnancy, I more closely resembled a blimp than a glowing yummy mummy.

Before I was diagnosed with preeclampsia, I had very little understanding of what it was. My only real point of reference was Lady Sybil from *Downton Abbey*, and without dropping too many spoilers, let's just say her experience of preeclampsia is not a positive one. Therefore, when the midwives routinely checked my wee, I never worried. Even when my legs were the same size from top to bottom, I had frequent headaches and started seeing stars, I still never worried. This was my first pregnancy and I told myself these were normal for the final trimester. Pregnancy hadn't been easy, so why would those final months be any different?

It's estimated that up to 10% of women will be diagnosed with preeclampsia in pregnancy, and when you think of how many women this will affect, it's unsurprising that midwives check for it routinely. But what is more surprising is that it is not discussed. If one in ten of us will get it, why don't we talk about it? I had little knowledge of preeclampsia when I was diagnosed, and therefore I wasn't worried. But I should have been, at least enough to take my symptoms more seriously. So, I hope by sharing these symptoms with you it doesn't frighten you, but just makes you more aware of what to look out for.

Preeclampsia usually occurs in the second half of pregnancy with symptoms beginning after 20 weeks. These symptoms include excessive swelling of hands, feet and face, which often is missed because most pregnant women hardly have the ankles of temple dancers! But in my case, my swelling covered my entire legs and face, so much so that I look back on photos of myself in my final months and genuinely don't recognise myself. If your face swells, then do push for another check. I also had swelling in my hands which didn't go away after birth, in fact, preeclampsia can occur after birth and continue for some time afterwards. It was weeks of sleeping in wrist supports before my fingers lost their sausageness after delivery.

The other symptom is headaches, and because I've always suffered with these, I didn't think twice about the migraines I began suffering with in my third trimester. But if these occur with any change of vision, do get it checked. I began seeing stars and dots; as I type, this sounds like an obvious problem, but how many women have truly never seen dots when they have stood up too quickly. I felt silly to mention this, as if I was being a drama queen, flagging normal things as problems. But if this experience has taught me anything, it's that there's no such thing as a silly question for your midwife!

I know now why it's important to associate these symptoms with preeclampsia and not just late pregnancy, because if monitored, preeclampsia can be a managed part of your pregnancy, however, if left it can be fatal to both mother and baby. And this is where the keen eye of a fabulous midwife saved both me and my baby.

I met a wonderfully powerful and forthright midwife during a routine check-up on the ward. She wasn't my usual midwife, just a member of staff on shift who came to check on me. By this point my headaches were getting worse, and the swelling meant I could barely walk. Instead of classing this as normal pregnancy, like I and many others had already done, this midwife marched across to the ward desk, and made a very determined (and may I add scary and loud!) phone call to the specialist. I heard her clearly demand that a doctor be sent to the ward immediately, and I don't blame them for following her assertive commands.

The midwife chased until I could be seen and oversaw all tests and ensured my results were rushed through. However, miraculously never made me feel frightened, simply supported. I was told to go home, await my results and relax. I wasn't worried as I was still weeks away from my due date and had only finished work that morning (I foolishly thought I'd given myself a few weeks to relax before baby... best laid plans of mice and men and all that!).

Within hours, I received a phone call to come up to the ward with my birth bag (definitely not packed at this point) and I was admitted to hospital that same evening. It was when in hospital that the nurses told me I would be induced that evening for both mine and my baby's safety. It was only at this moment did I realise that maybe all those symptoms were not normal, and that what was to follow certainly wasn't what I'd included in my mythical birth plan. So, at 36 + 5 weeks pregnant I was induced.

An induced labour comes with its own complications and additional pain. There is a great deal of research and impassioned views about the negative effects of an induced labour, and it's not that I disagree with these views. However, I didn't have the luxury of choice or strong opinions, I needed the baby out!

The one complication I will talk about, is that my wonderfully stubborn little boy, true to form, had made up his mind that he simply wasn't ready to be born. He was looking forward to a few more weeks in the comfort of my womb, and if he was going to be evicted in an untimely fashion, well he would leave kicking and screaming!

This isn't a piece about labour or a political expression about the pros and cons of induced labour. It's my experience before labour, and how preeclampsia changed my final weeks of pregnancy and my first few months of motherhood. The delivery of the baby is the only cure for preeclampsia, and even then, it doesn't disappear overnight. In fact, some women develop preeclampsia post-partum, therefore looking out for the symptoms is just as important post labour. I was fortunate to be seeing a physiotherapist (a detail which can be saved for a piece on the complications of birth!), who was able to treat my hands and help me regain better control in my hands and eventually reduce my swelling.

Having had preeclampsia with my first pregnancy increases my risk of developing it again in any future pregnancies. I'll be deemed high risk and closely monitored throughout, with every likelihood that my next pregnancy will end like my first. Does that worry me? Not at all. Forewarned is forearmed. This time, I know what to look out for and therefore how I treat myself will be different. No more working up to the very last possible week, forcing my bloated sausage legs into work clothes and to patrol playgrounds. And this time I will flag everything, whether I feel stupid or not! I won't be worried going on to that ward again (hopefully better prepared) because I know from experience that the midwives will do everything to keep me safe. And that wonderful woman who pushed my results through last time? I found out later that despite not being on shift the following day, she'd phoned the ward to check my results had come through and to check I was in hospital and safe. She later told me her own daughter had had similar symptoms with preeclampsia and so she'd used her prior knowledge to diagnose me, but she shouldn't have had to. I should have known about preeclampsia and taken my symptoms seriously myself.

May marks "Preeclampsia Awareness Day", a day that works to raise awareness of preeclampsia and improve research into it to reduce the impact it has on the lives of thousands of women and babies. Although not usually an ardent follower of "National [insert random celebration here] Day", this will certainly be one day that I do shout about in the hope that it helps even one more woman spot her symptoms and get the help she needs.

Tamara

Tamara has diabetes, endometriosis, and a wonderful adopted daughter. A supportive husband helped her on her journey through pain to find her family.

I am Tamara and I am 34 years old. I have spent most of my life living in Guernsey. I left the island at 18 to go to university and become a teacher, before returning and starting my teaching career. I then left the island again in 2010 before returning in 2015. I have been married for almost 5 years and have recently had a child placed with us through adoption.

I was diagnosed with Type 1 Diabetes at the age of 6 and at that age, the ability to have children was never discussed. When I got to 16/17 years old the diabetic team started discussing what would happen if I was ever to try and have children. I was never told I couldn't have children but that it would be more complicated with lots of different things to consider. Children though weren't even on my mind. I was more concerned about exams and going to University. While studying I met my (now ex) boyfriend and we were together for 8 years. During that time I had a pregnancy 'scare'. I had just started a new job in Guernsey and he was living and working for the government in the UK. He was supportive and was saying all the right things and as my contract was only until July the plan was I would move back to the UK. When I did a pregnancy test it came back negative. It didn't explain why I was constantly feeling sick, tired, getting lots of pain, and feeling like my stomach was going to explode but getting no monthly cycle. I went to the GP and explained my symptoms. About 3 weeks before the move back to England, I discovered it might be Endometriosis. My mum suffers from this condition and I was told it could be hereditary. As time went on things were getting a lot worse. If I had a period I would pass out, be sick and in so much pain, unable to move. This put a lot of pressure on my relationship and my ex would say things like "you're being stupid and get over it". After about a year and a half, I went to the doctors as whatever was happening was having a big impact on my life. Being in the UK however you never saw the same doctor so I had to repeat myself a few times. Eventually, I was referred to have more tests done in hospital. I was able to go private which only meant a 6-week wait instead of about 8 months. I had a laparoscopy where the surgeon found a large amount of Endometriosis which he burnt off. He also found I had cysts on the ovaries which were twisting. This was causing the severe pain. I was also put on codeine, diclofenac and anti-sickness to control any future pain. Unfortunately, after the surgery, although I said there was something wrong, I was sent home. After my mum arrived and saw the state I was in, I was taken straight to hospital where it was found my kidneys were starting to fail. By this point the relationship with my ex was almost non-existent, although we were due to get married 10 months later. My ex came to the follow-up appointment with me where the surgeon said he saw no reason why I couldn't have children but he recommended starting to try soon. That added more pressure and for the first time I started to think maybe I wouldn't be able to have children. I was only 24 years old. By that Christmas, the relationship was over and as my ex told me he had found someone else who 'was better at everything'. In my mind, this meant she was able to give him the family that he wanted. I met my now-husband a few months afterwards and after a year we moved in together and got engaged. I was very open with him about my concerns about not being able to have children and if this was the case I would understand if he wanted to leave and find someone else. He was fine with it and we both agreed if we really wanted children we would consider adoption. The side effects of the Endometriosis were still really bad and he will never let me forget the time he had just sat down to watch the new Transformers film when I sent him a text explaining I had passed out and couldn't move for the pain. He came home and sorted me out. I went back to see a GP who was shocked I had been taking Diclofenac by that point for almost 2 years as I should have never been on it that long. He took me off all medication. I noticed however that the pain was getting worse as the pressure on me at work was increasing. I was very stressed! We decided to move back to Guernsey after my now fiance was offered a job over here. We moved back, got married, and moved house twice in 6 weeks, it wasn't the right time to start a family so we didn't think much about it. I was back under the care of my old diabetic team who made it clear if I was to try for a baby I would be at an increased risk of miscarriage as my diabetes had not been controlled or monitored properly in the UK. In the 5 years I was there I saw a nurse once who it appeared needed to tick a box to say she had seen me so I could get my medication. After about a year of marriage, we decided we wanted to try for a baby. My sugars were better and the doctor put me on folic acid. We kept trying but nothing was happening. Every negative test was a blow and I would be disappointed but not show how I was really feeling. I would look for the slightest of change and then hope I would be pregnant. However, things were changing but not for the reasons we hoped for.

By this point my body was also starting to reject insulin and the word cysts were mentioned again. We discussed adoption and this was going to be the direction we went in if it didn't work out. After about a year of trying, I went to see the doctor and she referred me to a specialist.

While waiting for the appointment I had all the symptoms I could be pregnant. Around the time I was planning to do a test, I collapsed at work again in severe pain and bleeding. It could have been a miscarriage but we would never know. Once the appointment came around I had blood tests and scans and the specialist found I had a large number of cysts on my ovaries on both sides and I was booked in to have another Laparoscopy. They drilled into the ovaries and removed some cysts. This time he didn't see any Endometriosis.

By this point we had also contacted Guernsey Family Services and had been put on a pre-adoption course. This was around the time of the surgery, which went well and I was able to continue attending the course, although in a bit of pain. At the follow-up appointment the specialist said there was no reason why I couldn't carry a child but I would need to have IVF as I would not get pregnant without support. I was glad we had approached family services when we did. I think always having the feeling we wouldn't have children of our own made the news from the doctor not as bad as I knew we would have a child, just through different means. After the course, we were allocated a social worker who met with us regularly to fill in paperwork and write the report which would go to the panel. 9 months after first approaching Family Services we were approved to be adopters and it was now just the wait to be matched with a child. Our social worker was fantastic and kept us updated through face to face chats, phone calls and emails.

The wait seemed to go on forever and at times it was hard. The hardest part was everyone asking if I had any news. I got used to saying "no news yet but I'm not worried. It means they don't have to cover me at work yet." I kept management fully informed of everything that was happening and they were very supportive. Just after the COVID lockdown we were contacted about a child which we agreed to take on a foster to adopt placement. 48 hours after meeting her, she moved in. The last 5 weeks have been manic and I am sure we have been through the same experiences new parents have, even though she is 5. I would say 'we', but I think it is more me that is suffering from sleep deprivation and find it a little bit disconcerting waking up to find her staring at me at 6am in the morning and shouting down to my husband that I'm awake. He normally is up by 5am!! We've had tears and feeling like we don't know what we are doing and the panic of 'Oh My God she is going to hurt herself and we are going to be in so much trouble with social services.' Saying all that though adoption is not as scary as you think and I am glad my husband was so on board with the plan.

Everyone's journey to parenthood will be different and people will have different feelings about what route is best for them. For me, I didn't want to go down the IVF route. I have been lucky in that my husband has been so supportive and on board with the plans. If he hadn't of been however I wouldn't have blamed him. We approach everything as a partnership. The hardest part for me was all my siblings and cousins getting pregnant around the same time, the babies were all born within 5 months of each other, and it was emotional. It was only after I saw a baby scan come through to my mum's phone from my stepbrother, I cried. My mum and stepdad had been trying to hide the news from us, knowing how long we had been trying for a baby. It gets to a point where you can't hide those emotions anymore. Talking to people and family was the best thing to do because it made me realise that they understand and although they didn't tell me at the time, they had issues as well. One of my cousins was trying for 10 years before going down the IVF route and then had issues during the IVF. They now have a beautiful little girl. Just being honest with people was the best thing. When people at work asked when I was going to have a baby and asking if I was pregnant (I would bloat so much I looked as if I was 6 months pregnant) I would just say "We can't have children." The comments soon stopped. My colleagues were very supportive when they found out we were adopting. Although adoption for some people sounds daunting and scary, never rule it out. Guernsey Family Services have been amazing with their support and even though our little one is not biologically ours, we are a family.

A film we watched before she arrived was "Instant Family". It was hilarious and we now realise those things do happen sometimes, although we haven't set fire to anything and we haven't had any incidents with a tool. The message that comes across in the film is how you need a support network to get through the hard times. This is true, not just in adoption, but when you are trying so hard for a family of your own. You sometimes just need people to talk through things with and get all your emotions out there.

V.A.

This contributor talks candidly about the fact that actually, sometimes you can't just Talk About It. She calls her writing here 'The Sound of Silence' and I know it will resonate with several women who have thought about, and respectfully declined, contributing to this book.

I couldn't not contribute to this book. I remember my first reaction was to just pretend it was not being written because I could not face going down that hole again. Of course, you never forget and like anybody who has experienced grief, you expect and brace yourself for the occasional ebb and flow of sorrow but to knowingly go there, to plan to sit down and talk or write about it is a whole different story. It takes a lot of courage to expose your vulnerability and I admire all those women who have had the strength to do it. I am not there yet, I still find it terribly painful, even 5 years down the line. So, I will not write about my baby boy or going into labour or the funeral. I just wanted to write about Silence...

The Silence that follows the birth is quite crushing considering having a baby is all but quiet! It permeates the delivery room, pervades the hospital, and follows you into your home... It is palpable, you can almost touch it, taste it. It penetrates the walls and Silence comes along with a stillness that is eerie; people tiptoe around you, scared to hurt your feelings or say something that might make you cry, so they remain quiet or avoid you because they know that nothing can be said to soothe you. To some extent they are right, no word can provide comfort when you are in that bottomless pit, only time can heal.

I found that it felt like I was wearing ear defenders the few weeks that followed...sounds were muffled, lips would move but I would not care to join in conversations. Surprisingly enough though, while I found that my sense of hearing was taking the backseat, my sense of smell became more acute. Friends and families flooded us with flowers and each and every room had a bunch of flowers...while I floated sometimes aimlessly and restlessly in the house, those flowers reminded me how loved I was and that even if words were often not spoken, loved ones were there holding me up and helping me take a step at a time.

Flowers took a totally different dimension and meaning since then...particularly daffodils, the 'golden daffodils'...they were in bloom during that period. I must say that since, I often find myself re-reading William Wordsworth 'I wandered as lonely as a cloud'; his words strike a chord with me and I share his belief that there is something that unites us all, man and nature... and I would add 'the gone too soon' too. There is much comfort and solace to be derived from the thought that we are all connected in some shape or form, and I personally believe that this transcends death.

I wanted to hopefully be the voice of Silence, of all those women out there who still cannot speak about their loss because of various reasons. Silence can be so profound and deafeningly loud, and whatever your reasons are for not sharing your loss, you are not alone. Maybe, one day, in your own time you'll want to share. Maybe with time, all of us Survivors, will be able to find peace and and 'dance with the daffodils'

Recommended Reading

Aside from what may be mentioned in individual contributions, this is a list of what the ladies in this book have recommended.

Podcasts
Big Fat Negative Podcast - *Infertility and IVF*
Life After Miscarriage Podcast
Feathering the Empty Nest Podcast

Books
It's About Bloody Time. Period. by Emma Barnett
One and Only by Lauren Sandler - *Only children*
The Next Happy by Tracey Cleantis - *Letting go of the life you planned*
Living the Life Unexpected by Jody Day
No Matter What by Sally Donovan - *Adoption*
Love, Labour and Loss: Stillbirth and neonatal death by Jo Benson and Dawn Robinson
The Brink of Being by Julia Bueno
Miscarriage by Prof. Lesley Regan
A Bump In The Road by Elle Wright- *Fertility*

Online
The Gateway Women - *Online community for childless women*

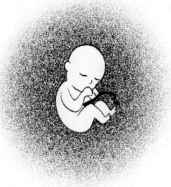

I hope you've enjoyed these Letters to Other Women. I know that everyone involved in this Lockdown Project wanted to share their story with the aim of supporting others, raising awareness and not letting anyone feel alone.

Thank you for letting us Talk About It.
For more information and for future projects, check out
Instagram: @LettersToOtherWomen

Notes, Reflections and Thoughts

If I Can Stop One Heart From Breaking

If I can stop one heart from breaking,
I shall not live in vain;
If I can ease one life the aching,
Or cool one pain,
Or help one lonely person
Into happiness again
I shall not live in vain.

Emily Dickinson

Acknowledgements

Of course this project wouldn't be complete without the contributions from the women in this book. Thank you all; your words mean a lot.

Thanks to Jozane and Luca from Book Printing UK, who helped create the physical book for us to read and smell. (Don't judge me, just sniff the book)

Thanks also to my husband Adam who has been with me on this journey of Making A Book from the beginning and has answered a tireless amount of questions.

And thank you, Wilf. I love you dude.